Clinical Handbook of Contact Dermatitis

Clinical Handbook of Contact Dermatitis

Diagnosis and Management by Body Region

Edited by

Robin Lewallen, MD
Adele Clark, PA-C
Steven R. Feldman, MD, PhD
Department of Dermatology
Wake Forest University School of Medicine
Winston-Salem, North Carolina, USA

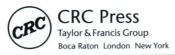

CRC Press
Taylor & Francis Group
Boca Raton London New York

CRC Press is an imprint of the
Taylor & Francis Group, an **informa** business

CRC Press
Taylor & Francis Group
6000 Broken Sound Parkway NW, Suite 300
Boca Raton, FL 33487-2742

© 2015 by Taylor & Francis Group, LLC
CRC Press is an imprint of Taylor & Francis Group, an Informa business

No claim to original U.S. Government works

Printed on acid-free paper
Version Date: 20140728

International Standard Book Number-13: 978-1-4822-3717-7 (Paperback)

This book contains information obtained from authentic and highly regarded sources. While all reasonable efforts have been made to publish reliable data and information, neither the author[s] nor the publisher can accept any legal responsibility or liability for any errors or omissions that may be made. The publishers wish to make clear that any views or opinions expressed in this book by individual editors, authors or contributors are personal to them and do not necessarily reflect the views/opinions of the publishers. The information or guidance contained in this book is intended for use by medical, scientific or health-care professionals and is provided strictly as a supplement to the medical or other professional's own judgement, their knowledge of the patient's medical history, relevant manufacturer's instructions and the appropriate best practice guidelines. Because of the rapid advances in medical science, any information or advice on dosages, procedures or diagnoses should be independently verified. The reader is strongly urge to consult the relevant national drug formulary and the drug companies' printed instructions, and their websites, before administering any of the drugs recommended in this book. This book does not indicate whether a particular treatment is appropriate or suitable for a particular individual. Ultimately it is the sole responsibility of the medical professional to make his or her own professional judgements, so as to advise and treat patients appropriately. The authors and publishers have also attempted to trace the copyright holders of all material reproduced in this publication and apologize to copyright holders if permission to publish in this form has not been obtained. If any copyright material has not been acknowledged please write and let us know so we may rectify in any future reprint.

Except as permitted under U.S. Copyright Law, no part of this book may be reprinted, reproduced, transmitted, or utilized in any form by any electronic, mechanical, or other means, now known or hereafter invented, including photocopying, microfilming, and recording, or in any information storage or retrieval system, without written permission from the publishers.

For permission to photocopy or use material electronically from this work, please access www.copyright.com (http://www.copyright.com/) or contact the Copyright Clearance Center, Inc. (CCC), 222 Rosewood Drive, Danvers, MA 01923, 978-750-8400. CCC is a not-for-profit organization that provides licenses and registration for a variety of users. For organizations that have been granted a photocopy license by the CCC, a separate system of payment has been arranged.

Trademark Notice: Product or corporate names may be trademarks or registered trademarks, and are used only for identification and explanation without intent to infringe.

Library of Congress Cataloging-in-Publication Data

Clinical handbook of contact dermatitis : diagnosis and management by body region / editors, Robin Lewallen, Adele Clark, Steven R. Feldman.
    p. ; cm.
Includes bibliographical references and index.
ISBN 978-1-4822-3717-7 (pbk. : alk. paper)
I. Lewallen, Robin, editor. II. Clark, Adele, 1956- , editor. III. Feldman, Steven R., editor.
[DNLM: 1. Dermatitis, Contact--diagnosis. 2. Dermatitis, Contact--therapy. WR 175]

RL244
616.5'1--dc23   2014028246

Visit the Taylor & Francis Web site at
http://www.taylorandfrancis.com

and the CRC Press Web site at
http://www.crcpress.com

Table of Contents

Acknowledgments

This text is partially comprised of articles that have been previously published, although the content has been edited and updated. We would like to extend special recognition to Dr. Matthew Zirwas of Ohio State University Wexner Medical Center for his help with the original publications.

Members of staff at the Department of Dermatology, Wake Forest University School of Medicine, very kindly contributed to this text: Michael Chung, BS; Monica Huynh, BA; Farah Moustafa, BS; Courtney Orscheln, MD; and Laura Sandoval, DO. Michael P. Sheehan, MD, of Indiana University, also kindly contributed to the text.

CHAPTER 1

Introduction to contact dermatitis

Robin Lewallen and Steven R. Feldman

Contact dermatitis is a common skin condition frequently seen by physicians. It affects approximately 20% of people in the United States. It is responsible for 70 to 80% of all reported occupational skin diseases, and it is a frequent chief complaint of clinic visits.[1] There are two main types of contact dermatitis: irritant contact dermatitis and allergic contact dermatitis. Irritant contact dermatitis (ICD) is far more frequent than allergic contact dermatitis (ACD). While the clinical appearance may be similar, allergic contact dermatitis differs from irritant dermatitis in many ways (Table 1.1).

Table 1.1 – Allergic versus irritant contact dermatitis

	Allergic contact dermatitis	Irritant contact dermatitis
Definition	An acquired inflammatory response to an allergen that occurs only in individuals who have been sensitized to the allergen	A nonspecific immune reaction of the skin to a substance that results in a skin eruption in any individual exposed to a high enough concentration
Molecular mechanism	Cell-mediated hypersensitivity through Langerhans cells and CD4+ T cells after contact with a specific allergen (delayed Type IV hypersensitivity reaction)	Skin barrier disruption and cellular damage of the keratinocyte membrane from contact when an irritant activates the innate immune system
Time between exposure and cutaneous manifestation	Hours to days	Within minutes to several hours
Body location	Scalp is uncommon	Hands and face are common
Symptoms	Itching	Pain and burning

Factors that alter severity of reaction	Concentration of allergen and length of exposure Atopic patients are reported to be less likely to have ACD	Dry skin and thicker skin reacts less severely Atopic patients react more severely due to reduced barrier function
Common allergens/irritants	Top 10 allergens from patch test results[2]: nickel sulfate, balsam of Peru (*Myroxylon pereirae*), fragrance mix, quaternium-15, neomycin sulfate, bacitracin, formaldehyde, cobalt chloride, methyldibromo glutaronitrile, and p-phenylenediamine	Top irritants[3,4]: low humidity, heat, water, detergents, solvents, oils, heat and sweating, dust and fibers, acids, and alkalis
Histology	Acute: epidermal spongiosis with superficial dermal edema, eosinophils, and mild perivascular lymphocytic infiltrate in the upper dermis; vesicles can contain neutrophils Chronic: psoriasiform changes	Varies depending on the severity and chronicity of exposure Low concentrations: mimics acute ACD High concentrations: epidermal necrosis, which can be full thickness with balloon degeneration
Testing	Patch test Photopatch test Provocative use test	None

The list of allergens that cause ACD continues to grow. There are over 3,500 environmental contact allergens reported in the literature.[5] Exposure to a particular allergen can occur for years before developing a delayed hypersensitivity immune response. After sensitization occurs, subsequent exposure to the allergen may result in ACD even if used in small concentrations.[6] Poison ivy (urushiol) is another common allergen but is not included in typical testing or in the frequency results by the North American Contact Dermatitis Group (NACDG). Topical medications are a common cause of contact dermatitis, including antibiotics (58%), corticosteroids (30%), and anesthetics (6%). This generates a conundrum when selecting treatments for contact dermatitis, as upwards of 30% of patients with a medication allergy had a positive patch test to a topical corticosteroid, either the steroid or the vehicle.[7] Many of the products that are used on a daily basis contain one or more potential allergens (Table 1.2).

While ACD is a specific reaction to an allergen that occurs only in sensitized individuals, ICD can occur in anyone exposed to an irritant at a high concentration or for a significant length of time. There are many substances that can disrupt the skin's barrier and activate the innate immune response. Occupational dermatitis, which is in large part caused by irritant dermatitis, costs up to $1 billion annually from medical bills, medications, worker's compensation, and lost work hours.[8]

Table 1.2 – Products containing common allergens

Product	Allergen
Metals	Nickel, cobalt, sodium gold thiosulfate, potassium dichromate
Fragrance	Balsam of Peru (*Myroxylon pereirae*), ylang-ylang oil, jasmine Fragrance mix I (cinnamic aldehyde, cinnamyl alcohol, hydroxycitronellal, isoeugenol, eugenol, oak moss absolute, α-amyl cinnamic aldehyde, geraniol) Fragrance mix II (Lyral®, citral, farnesol, citronellol, hexyl cinnamic aldehyde, coumarin)
Rubber accelerators and latex	Carba mix, mercaptobenzothiazole (MBT), thiuram mix, mercapto mix, black rubber mix, mixed dialkyl thioureas
Leather	Tanning solutions: potassium dichromate
	Leather gloves and watch bands: p-tert-butylphenol formaldehyde resin
Adhesives	Colophony, ethylenediamine dihydrochloride, epoxy resin, p-tert-butylphenol formaldehyde resin, ethylacrylate, methyl methacrylate
Nails	Nail polish: tosylamide formaldehyde resin
	Artificial nail glue: ethyl acrylate, methyl methacrylate
Hair	Shampoos: quaternium-15, methyldibromo glutaronitrile/phenoxyethanol, cocamidopropyl betaine/amidoamine, imidazolidinyl urea, cocamide DEA, methylchloroisothiazolinone/methylisothiazolinone (MCI/MI), fragrances
	Permanent wave solutions: glyceryl thioglycolate
	Hair dyes: p-phenylenediamine (PPD), cobalt
Clothing and textiles	Dyes: disperse blue 106 and 124 (increased amounts found in dark clothing)
	Permanent press clothing (used most often to provide wrinkle resistance in cotton, rayon, and cotton polyester blends, and not often used in wool, nylon, and silk fabrics): ethylenurea melamine-formaldehyde, dimethylol dihydroxyethyleneurea
	Footwear: mercaptobenzothiazole (MBT), potassium dichromate, and colophony

Cosmetics and personal care products	Fragrances and preservatives: propylene glycol, phenylenediamine, lanolin alcohol, amidoamine, benzophenone, chloroxylenol, alpha tocopherol, cocamidopropyl betaine, cocamide DEA, ylang-ylang oil, paraben mix, methyldibromo glutaronitrile/phenoxyethanol, iodopropynyl butylcarbamate, 2-bromo-2-nitropropane-1,3-diol (Bronopol®)
Preservatives	Formaldehyde-releasing preservatives: quaternium-15, formaldehyde, diazolidinyl urea, imidazolidinyl urea, DMDM hydantoin, 2-bromo-2-nitropropane-1,3 diol (Bronopol®), ethylene urea/melamine formaldehyde, dimethylol, dihydroxyethyleneurea
	Other preservatives: methylchloroisothiozolinene, paraben mix, methyldibromo glutaronitril, thimerosal, methydibromo glutaronitrite/phenoxyethanol, iodopropynyl butylcarbamate, tosylamide formaldehyde resin, phenoxyethanol, benzalkonium chloride, glutaral
Sunscreen	Fragrances and preservatives (see above) Photocontact: benzophenone-3/oxybenzone, cinnamic aldehyde
Topical medications	Fragrances and preservatives (see above) Antibiotics: neomycin sulfate, bacitracin
	Corticosteroids: tixocortol-21-pivalate (Class A), budesonide (Class B), desoximetasone (Class C), and hydrocortisone-17 butyrate (Class D)
	Anesthetics, including medications for hemorrhoids, teething, cold sores, canker sores: lidocaine, benzocaine
	Antihistamines: ethylenediamine dihydrochloride
	Ophthalmic drops and vaccines: thimerosal (preservative)
	Antabuse: thiuram mix
	Vehicles and emulsifiers: colophony, lanolin, propylene glycol, sorbitan sesquioleate
Temporary Tattoos (black henna)	p-Phenylenediamine (PPD)
Emollients	Fragrances and preservatives (see above) Lanolin (wool alcohol), methylchloroisothiozolinone/methylisothiazolinone (MCI/MI) in Eucerin®

Source: Adapted from References 2 and 7.

Irritant dermatitis is more common in women than men. ICD is also much more common in certain locations on the body, such as the hands and face, as these areas are frequently exposed to irritants. Some of the most commonly implicated irritants include low humidity, heat, metals, paper, tools, fibers/fabrics, plastics, dust, woods, rubber, jewelry, seasonal environment, fiberglass, and hearing aids.[4] In many cases the mechanism, such as friction and drying, are just as important in causing ICD as the physical irritant.

Our goal is to provide a regional approach to contact dermatitis with the hope of making this vast subject area more approachable and clinically useful. Any topical skin product containing a variety of fragrances, preservatives, and other additives, needs to be considered as a potential allergen in all cases of contact dermatitis. However there are also a number of less common materials and products that need to be considered as an allergy source. We use a systematic approach to discuss some of the most common allergens and irritants in a given body location. We also provide guidance in diagnosis and treatment options including topical medications and patch testing (see Chapters 12 and 13 for additional information).

References

1. Rietschel RL, Mathias CG, Fowler Jr JF, et al. 2002. Relationship of occupation to contact dermatitis: Evaluation in patients tested from 1998 to 2000. *Am J Contact Dermat* 13:170–176.
2. Zug KA, Warshaw EM, Fowler JF Jr, Maibach HI, Belsito DL, Pratt MD, Sasseville D, et al. 2009. Patch-test results of the North American Contact Dermatitis Group 2005–2006. *Dermatitis* 20(3):149–160.
3. Slodownik D, Lee A, Nixon R. 2008. Irritant contact dermatitis: A review. *Australas J Dermatol* 49(1):1–9.
4. Morris-Jones R, Robertson SJ, Ross JS, White IR, McFadden JP, Rycroft RJ. 2002. Dermatitis caused by physical irritants. *Br J Dermatol* 147(2):270–275.
5. Mortz, CG, Andersen, KE. 2008. New aspects in allergic contact dermatitis. *Current Opinion in Allergy and Clinical Immunology* 8(5):428–432.
6. James WD, Berger TG, Elston D, eds. 2010. *Andrews' Diseases of the Skin: Clinical Dermatology*, 11th edition. Philadelphia: WB Sanders.
7. Spring S, Pratt M, Chaplin A. 2012. Contact dermatitis to topical medicaments: A retrospective chart review from the Ottawa Hospital Patch Test Clinic. *Dermatitis* 23(5):210–213.
8. Cohen DE. 2000. *Occupational dermatoses*. In: Harris RL, ed. *Patty's Industrial Hygiene*, 5th edition, pp. 165–210. New York: John Wiley.

CHAPTER 2
Scalp

Monica Huynh, Michael P. Sheehan, Michael Chung,
Matthew Zirwas, and Steven R. Feldman

Although the scalp is commonly exposed to many articles and products containing known allergens, isolated scalp dermatitis due to contact dermatitis is relatively uncommon. This appears to be primarily due to a topographical property innate to the scalp. The thicker scalp skin, with abundant pilosebaceous units and a relative absence of rhytids or crevices, is the ideal barrier against contact dermatitis. In contrast, the eyelids are on the other end of the spectrum, with very thin skin and many folds that retain substances, increasing time exposure and resulting in more severe reactions. For these reasons, contact dermatitis is unlikely to be at the top of the differential diagnosis for isolated scalp dermatitis. Even in cases where an aggressive allergen is present, the scalp is often not affected or only minimally affected, despite significant involvement of the face, ears and/or neck.[1] It is often more useful to talk about "scalp-applied" irritants and allergens rather than isolated scalp contact dermatitis.

Presentation

Potential allergens involved in scalp dermatitis have been reviewed. Patients with documented scalp dermatitis who underwent patch testing showed that hair dyes, hair cleansing products, and medicaments combined for nearly two-thirds of the positive patch test reactions.[2] Unfortunately, the study was not designed to assess the relevance of these positive patch tests. Looking at the pattern of dermatitis is helpful when trying to determine which allergen is involved (Table 2.1).

Regional consideration of the scalp in contact dermatitis requires the clinician to ask two important questions. First, "Is there a primary dermatitis involving the scalp?" As with any anatomical region, geometric areas of dermatitis are nearly pathognomonic for contact dermatitis. On the scalp, this may take the form of jewelry, such as nickel hairpins, clasps, or other decorative items. Curling irons and straighteners may also be a source of allergen exposure. These products most often cause problems in nickel-sensitive patients.[3] Bands of dermatitis that span the forehead, encircle the head, and/or affect the helices of the ears are suggestive of head accessories with leather or rubber parts, such as in hat bands or hat linings (Figure 2.1).[4] With such distribution, exposure to adhesive tapes used to fix wigs to the scalp should also be considered.[5]

Second, "Is there a primary dermatitis suggestive of a scalp applied allergen?" Allergic reactions to hair products are not largely restricted to the scalp and often

Table 2.1 – Scalp dermatitis—allergens with patterns

Agent	Allergen	Pattern
Headband, bathing cap, hairnet, hats	Leather or rubber	Linear rash across forehead Encircles head May involve ears
Wigs	Adhesives	Encircles head
Bobby pins, hair pins	Nickel	Discrete Corresponds with shape of offending agent
Wash-out products including shampoos and conditioners	Quaternium-15, methyldibromo glutaronitrile, phenoxyethanol, fragrance, MCI/MI, cocamidopropyl betaine	Rinse-off pattern Patchy distribution
Hair dyes	PPD	Acute edematous dermatitis
Permanent wave solutions	Glyceryl thioglycolate	Acute edematous dermatitis
Leave-in styling aids (mousse, gels, pomades, hairspray)	Fragrances, preservatives, acrylates	Chronic dermatitis with episodic flairs Hairspray can cause a dermatitis at the temples adjacent to the scalp

Note: MCI/MI = Methylchloroisothiazolinone/Methylisothiazolinone; PPD = p-Phenylenediamine

involve the face, eyelids, ears, and neck; a high degree of suspicion is critical to the diagnosis. The rinse-off or drip pattern sign is a clinically useful clue to suggest a scalp-applied allergen (Figure 2.2). This appears as a well-demarcated and relatively linear streaking dermatitis involving the pre-auricular face and lateral neck. In patients with classic rinse-off pattern of dermatitis, personal hair care products should be considered.[2] The most important potential allergens in shampoos and conditioners are fragrances, cocamidopropyl betaine (CAPB), and preservatives including quaternium-15.[6] CAPB is of particular interest and is contained in many shampoos, including those marketed as "no tears" products for infants and young children. Two somewhat unique patterns have been observed with CAPB sensitivity: chronic scalp pruritus and flaking, and a chronic dermatitis with episodic flares.[2]

Hair dye is a scalp-applied allergen that needs to be considered. In one study, hair dye was the most common cause of scalp dermatitis.[2] Paraphenylenediamine (PPD) is a frequently used oxidative colorant. In 2006 and 2007, it was reported that PPD contact allergy had increased significantly in the general population and, in 2006,

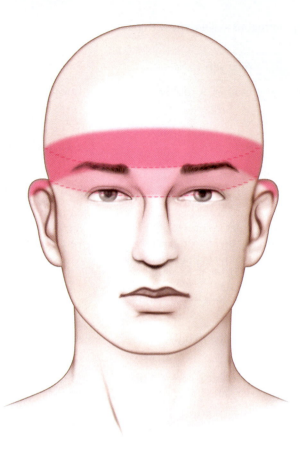

Figure 2.1 – Contact dermatitis due to head accessories.

PPD was named Contact Allergen of the Year by the American Contact Dermatitis Society.[7] In PPD-sensitive patients, there is often a robust acute dermatitis involving the face, eyelids, and neck, with only minimal scalp involvement (Figure 2.3).

An emerging allergen frequently applied to the scalp is *Melaleuca alternifolia*, commonly known as tea tree oil. Recent popularity is due in part to reports showing efficacy in the treatment of seborrheic dermatitis.[8] As with any potential contact allergen, *Melaleuca* sensitization and irritation is increased when exposure to inflamed and damaged skin occurs. Clinicians should consider this allergen in patients with recalcitrant, worsening, or flaring seborrheic dermatitis or sebopsoriasis. In this setting, asking the patient about the use of "natural" or over-the-counter remedies may lead to the discovery of *Melaleuca* exposure.

Minoxidil may be the most frequent cause of scalp dermatitis medicamentosa.[1] Although irritant contact dermatitis is the most frequent reported outcome of topical use of minoxidil, there are reports of allergic contact dermatitis on the scalp. A pustular eruption of the scalp has also been reported.[9,10]

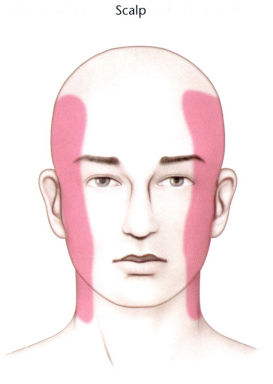

Figure 2.2 – Rinse-off pattern due to shampoo, conditioner, and other rinse-off products.

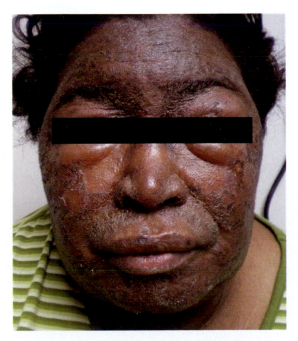

FIGURE 2.3 – Acute dermatitis from PPD-containing hair dye.

Table 2.2 – Minimally or hypoallergenic scalp products

Product	Allergen
Loprox Shampoo	None
Clobex Shampoo	Cocamidopropyl betaine
DHS Tar Shampoo (Fragrance Free)	None
Free and Clear Shampoo	None
RID Lice Removal Shampoo	Fragrance
California Baby Supersensitive Shampoo and Bodywash	Parabens
Neutrogena T/Sal Shampoo	Cocamidopropyl betaine

Recommendations

Management of suspected contact dermatitis of the scalp should include patch testing. However, an empiric trial of hypoallergenic products can be performed. Table 2.2 highlights some useful scalp products that are minimally or hypoallergenic.

References

1. Wolverton SE. 2013. *Comprehensive Dermatologic Drug Therapy*, 3rd edition. Philadelphia: Saunders.
2. Hillen U, Grabbe S, Uter W. 2007. Patch test results in patients with scalp dermatitis: Analysis of data of the Information Network of Departments of Dermatology. *Contact Dermatitis* 56:87–93.
3. Thyssen JP, Jensen P, Johansen JD, Menné T. 2009. Contact dermatitis caused by nickel release from hair clasps purchased in a country covered by the EU Nickel Directive. *Contact Dermatitis* 60(3):180–181.
4. Rietschel RL, Fowler JF, Fisher AA. 2001. *Fisher's Contact Dermatitis*, 5th edition. Philadelphia: Lippincott Williams & Wilkins.
5. Torchia D, Giorgini S, Gola M, Francalanci S. 2008. Allergic contact dermatitis from 2-ethylhexyl acrylate contained in a wig-fixing adhesive tape and its 'incidental' therapeutic effect on alopecia areata. *Contact Dermatitis* 58(3): 170–171.
6. Zirwas M, Moennich J. 2009. Shampoo. *Dermatitis* 20(2):106–110.
7. Krasteva M, Bons B, Ryan C, Gerberick GF. 2009. Consumer allergy to oxidative hair coloring products: Epidemiologic data in the literature. *Dermatitis* 20(3):123–141.
8. Satchell A, Sauralen AB, Barnetson R. 2002. Treatment of dandruff with 5% tea tree oil shampoo. *Journal of the American Academy of Dermatology* 47(6):852–858.

9. Friedman E, Friedman P, Cohen D, Washenik K. 2002. Allergic contact dermatitis to topical minoxidil solution: Etiology and treatment. *Journal of the American Academy of Dermatology* 406(2):309–312.
10. Rodríguez-Martin M, Sáez-Rodríguez M, Carnerero-Rodríguez A, Cabrera de Paz R, Sidro-Sarto M, Pérez-Robayna N, et al. 2007. Pustular allergic contact dermatitis from topical minoxidil 5%. *Journal of the European Academy of Dermatology & Venereology* 21(5):701–702.

CHAPTER 3
Face

Monica Huynh, Michael P. Sheehan, Michael Chung,
Matthew Zirwas, and Steven R. Feldman

Introduction

The face is widely exposed to the surrounding environment and is also a region that comes into frequent contact with the hands. As a result, contact dermatitis presenting on the face may be from a causative agent that had direct, indirect, or airborne contact. The face is also the most common site of photocontact dermatitis.[1] Therefore, the face is a highly complex region and can be difficult to assess. Paying close attention to characteristic patterns may provide clues to identifying the specific allergen or irritant.

Presentation

Facial contact dermatitis has a fairly well defined group of frequent offending allergens. Using a regional approach helps simplify this list into three main categories: scalp dermatitis, aerosolized allergens, and directly applied facial allergens/irritants (Table 3.1).

Table 3.1 – Useful product/allergens and patterns

Scalp-applied allergens (refer to Chapter 2 for complete list)	
Shampoos, conditioners, hair dye	Periphery of the face (pre-auricular, submental, and mandibular region), rinse-off pattern
Aeroallergens	
Fragrance, plant allergens, aerosols, animal dander, dust mites, pollen	Facial dermatitis, cutoff at shirt collar
Face-applied allergens	
Cosmetic products (makeup)	Bilateral, centralized (forehead, cheeks, chin), patchy/diffuse
Wash-out products (soaps)	Bilateral, centralized (forehead, cheeks, chin), patchy/diffuse

Table 3.1 – *(Continued)*

Leave-in products (lotions, sunscreens)	Bilateral, diffuse distribution
Cell phone (nickel or chromate)	Mid-to-lower cheek of lateral face, unilateral, bilateral if simultaneous use of two cell phones.
Eyewear (eyeglasses, sunglasses)	Bilateral, symmetrical, linear rash, corresponds to shape of eyewear, below eyes on upper cheeks
Scuba diver face masks	Bilateral, symmetrical, corresponds to shape of mask
Rubber cosmetic sponge	Patchy distribution, asymmetrical

The term *aerosolized contact allergens* (*aeroallergens*) should not be restricted to such things as animal dander, dust mites, and pollens, which more frequently drive Type I hypersensitivity reactions. Aeroallergens also include fragrances (Figures 3.1 and 3.2), plant allergens, and things that become temporarily aerosolized during repair or manufacturing processes. Aeroallergens have been classically reported to present as facial dermatitis with a distinct cutoff along the shirt collar. Aeroallergens are also sometimes contributors to a phototoxic or photoallergic reaction. Sparing under the chin or behind the ears is a clue to photo-exacerbation. Patients with

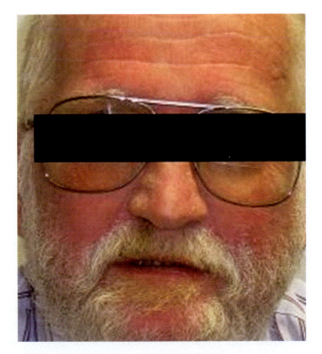

Figure 3.1 – Dermatitis due to fragrance (aeroallergen).

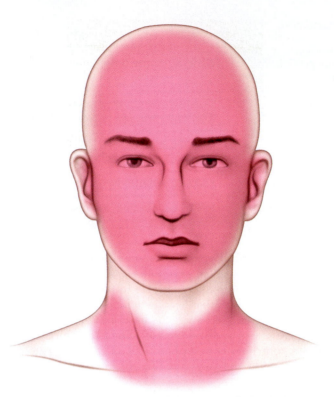

Figure 3.2 – Dermatitis due to fragrance (aeroallergen).

aeroallergen-driven facial dermatitis frequently have an underlying atopy. The "head-light" sign, which refers to the presence of facial dermatitis that dramatically spares the nose, may be useful clinically to suggest such patients (Figure 3.3).[2] It has been reported in patients with atopic dermatitis and neurodermatitis.

In a study performed by the North American Contact Dermatitis Group, females more frequently presented with facial contact dermatitis secondary to cosmetic-associated allergens.[3] Common sources among both females and males include moisturizers, sunscreens, hair products, and fragrances.[1,3] In general, cosmetic-related dermatitis favors a bilateral facial distribution. It is often patchy and diffuse. Predilection for the periphery of the face involving the pre-auricular, submental, and mandibular region should direct consideration toward scalp-applied allergens, such as shampoos, conditioners, and hair dyes, as well as wash-off products such as facial cleansers (Figure 3.4). This sign was introduced in Chapter 2 and is known as a rinse-off pattern. A predominantly central facial distribution (forehead, cheeks, and chin) suggests makeup, moisturizers, or jewelry (Figure 3.5).

A unilateral rash with patchy distribution along the mid-to-lower cheek of the lateral face is suggestive of a nickel or chromate allergy from cell phones (Figures 3.6 and 3.7).[4,5] An individual with symmetrical contact dermatitis due to simultaneous use of two cell phones was recently reported.[7]

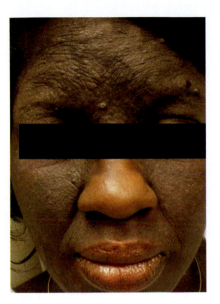

Figure 3.3 – Headlight sign: facial dermatitis that spares the nose.

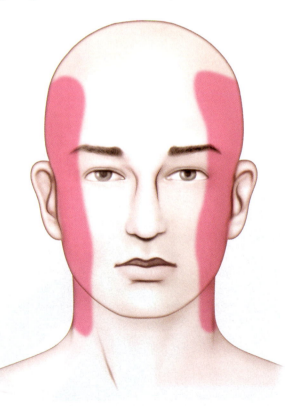

Figure 3.4 – Rinse-off pattern due to scalp-applied allergens and wash-out products.

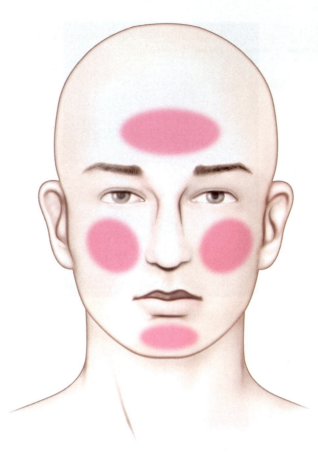

Figure 3.5 – Contact dermatitis due to makeup and moisturizer.

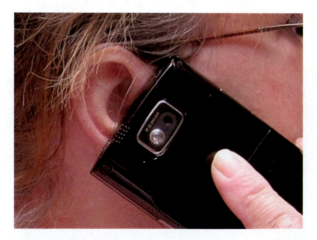

Figure 3.6 – Nickel or chromate allergy from cell phones.

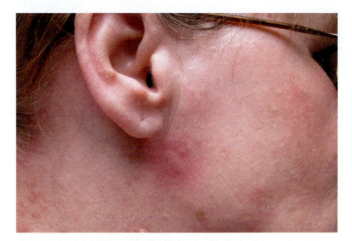

Figure 3.7 – Nickel or chromate allergy from cell phones.

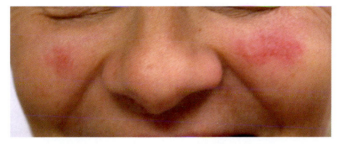

Figure 3.8 – Contact dermatitis due to nickel in eyewear. (Reproduced by courtesy of Courtney Orscheln.)

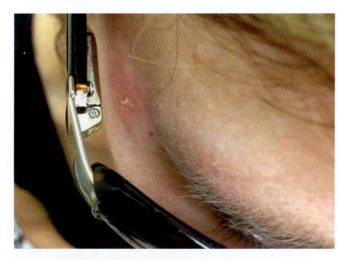

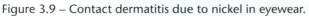
Figure 3.9 – Contact dermatitis due to nickel in eyewear.

Other potential nickel sources should be considered, such as eyewear. A bilateral rash on the upper cheek where the lower rims of eyewear potentially make contact with the skin is suggestive of an allergy to worn-out metal in eyewear (Figures 3.8 and 3.9).[1,6]

Rubber is another common cause of contact dermatitis, and rubber-induced rashes often present according to the shape of the offending object. Scuba diver face masks and swimming goggles produce a bilateral, symmetrical pattern that follows the outline of the product.[1] Rubber cosmetic sponges will cause a patchy distribution with an asymmetrical pattern, but may vary depending on the patient.[1]

References

1. Rietschel RL, Fowler JF, Fisher AA. 2001. *Fisher's Contact Dermatitis*, 5th edition. Philadelphia: Lippincott Williams & Wilkins.
2. Bender B, Prestia AE, Lynfield YL. The headlight sign in neurodermatitis. 1969. *Cutis* 5:1406–1408.
3. Castanedo-Tardan MP, Zug KA. 2009. Patterns of cosmetic contact allergy. *Dermatologic Clinics* 27(3):265–230.
4. Rajpara A, Feldman SR. 2010. Cell phone allergic contact dermatitis: Case report and review. *Dermatology Online Journal* 16(6):9.
5. Seishima M, Oyama Z, Oda, M. 2003. Cellular phone dermatitis with chromate allergy. *Dermatology* 207(1):48.
6. Scott K, Levender M, Feldman SR. 2010. Eyeglass allergic contact dermatitis. *Dermatology Online Journal* 16(9):11.
7. Ozkaya E. 2011. Bilateral symmetrical contact dermatitis on the face and outer thighs from the simultaneous use of two mobile phones. *Dermatitis* 22(2):116–118.

CHAPTER 4

Eyelids

Monica Huynh, Michael P. Sheehan, Michael Chung,
Matthew Zirwas, and Steven R. Feldman

Introduction

The eyelids are one of the most sensitive regions of the body, making them very susceptible to contact dermatitis. This may be explained by two major theories. The skin of the eyelids is quite thin (0.55 mm) compared to other sites on the face (2.0 mm); this suggests the eyelids would be more susceptible to damage and irritation.[1,2] The other theory focuses on the sphincter function of the orbicularis oculi. The accordion-like movement of the upper eyelid during blinking may lead to potential allergens becoming trapped and retained between the folded skin when the eye is open.[3] This would result in prolonged exposure. Regardless, the eyelids are more susceptible to both irritant and allergic contact dermatitis.

Presentation

Similar to the face, the eyelid region can be more easily approached by considering categories of allergen exposure. The five major categories are scalp-applied allergens, aeroallergens, directly contacted allergens, ectopic allergens, and inadvertent allergens. The first two categories have been covered in Chapters 2 and 3 on the scalp and face. We will consider the latter three further. Directly applied allergens include anything directly applied or exposed to the eyelid. This list is nearly endless and includes a myriad of cosmetics, cleansers, and ophthalmic medicaments. The most common allergens in this category are fragrances, preservatives, and nickel.[4,5] Nickel can be found as an ingredient or contaminate in personal care products such as makeup, but it is also found frequently in applicators.[6] These applicators may also be a source of rubber or black dye (p-paraphenylenediamine) exposure. A predominance of the lower eyelids with a "run-off" or "drip" pattern should raise suspicion of ophthalmic solutions (Figure 4.1).[3] Ophthalmic medications may contain potentially irritating and sensitizing preservatives, such as benzalkonium chloride, thimerosal (merthiolate), chlorobutanol, chlorohexidine, or phenylmercuric.[2] Topical medicaments such as antibiotics and steroids should also be considered. Finally, this category also includes things such as swim goggles, binocular or telescope eyepieces, and eye patches (Figure 4.2). These objects often cause a characteristic dermatitis that mimics their use. Figure 4.3 shows unilateral eyelid dermatitis in a medical technician student who used a monocular microscope with a rubber

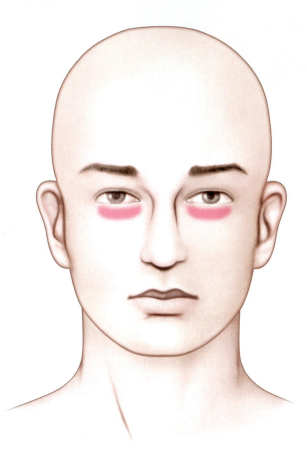

Figure 4.1 – Lower eyelid dermatitis due to ophthalmic medicaments.

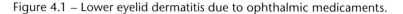

eyepiece. A similar unilateral eyelid dermatitis has also been seen in gastroenterologists who develop contact dermatitis to the glutaraldehyde used to cleanse colonoscopy and endoscopy scopes.

The category of ectopic allergens is an interesting one. The term is most often used when talking about eyelid dermatitis in relationship to gold.[7] It refers to the allergen source being removed or at an ectopic site from the dermatitis. Typically this can be from a gold ring on the finger. The situation may be somewhat perplexing in that patients frequently do not have a reaction to the allergen on the finger. The explanation for this seems to be that gold is released from the allergen source and transferred to the eyelid in the presence of sweat and abrasive particles such as titanium dioxide, a physical sunscreen and common ingredient in cosmetics.[7] Data from the North American Contact Dermatitis Group (NACDG) published in *Dermatitis* on isolated eyelid contact dermatitis revealed that gold was the most frequently encountered allergen producing a positive patch test.[4]

The "inadvertent" allergens are an easily forgotten but important cause of eyelid dermatitis. The eyelids are frequently rubbed and touched, which leads to transfer

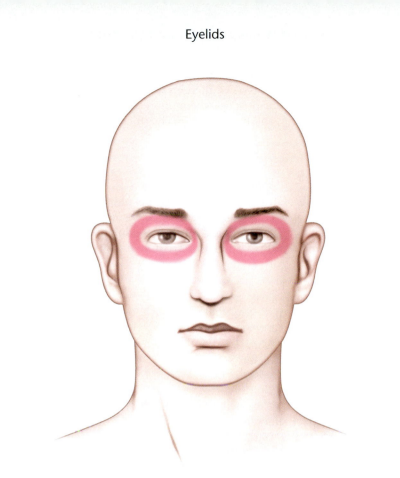

Figure 4.2 – Annular dermatitis due to goggles, binoculars, and other eyepieces.

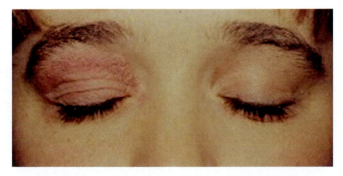

Figure 4.3 – Unilateral eyelid dermatitis as seen on a medical technician student using a monocular microscope with a rubber eyepiece.

of substances from the hands. In this manner, the eyelids may be exposed to a multitude of potential allergens. This type of allergen spread often appears as an isolated, asymmetric upper eyelid dermatitis. Some common sources include hand sanitizer, hand soap, hand moisturizer, and nail polish.[2,3] The thicker skin of the hands is often spared.

Recommendations

When allergic contact dermatitis of the eyelid is suspected, empiric use of minimally or hypoallergenic scalp-applied products, cleansers, cosmetics, and topical medications and products may be helpful. Topical immunomodulators such as topical tacrolimus could also be considered (Chapter 13, "Treatment Considerations").

References

1. Castanedo-Tardan MP, Zug KA. 2009. Patterns of cosmetic contact allergy. *Dermatologic Clinic* 27(3):265–230.
2. Rietschel RL, Fowler JF, Fisher AA. 2001. *Fisher's Contact Dermatitis*, 5th edition. Philadelphia: Lippincott Williams & Wilkins.
3. Wolverton, SE. 2013. *Comprehensive Dermatologic Drug Therapy*, 3rd edition, chapter 53. Philadelphia: Saunders.
4. Rietschel RL, Warshaw EM, Sasseville D, Fowler JF, DeLeo VA, Belsito DV, et al. 2007. Common contact allergens associated with eyelid dermatitis: Data from the North American Contact Dermatitis Group 2003–2004 Study Period. *Dermatitis* 18(2):78–81.
5. Valsecchi R, Imberti D, Martino D, et al. 1992. Eyelid dermatitis: An evaluation of 150 patients. *Contact Dermatitis* 27:143–147.
6. Henke U, Boehncke WH. Eyelid dermatitis caused by an eyelash former. *Contact Dermatitis* 53(4):237.
7. Nedorost S, Wagman A. 2005. Positive patch-test reactions to gold: Patients' perception of relevance and the role of titanium dioxide in cosmetics. *Dermatitis* 16(2):67–70.

CHAPTER 5

Mouth, lips, and perioral region

Michael P. Sheehan, Monica Huynh, Michael Chung, Matthew Zirwas, and Steven R. Feldman

Introduction

The oral region of the face is unique, with three different epithelial zones: the cutaneous lips, the vermillion, and the mucosa of the oral cavity. The skin of the cutaneous vermillion is similar to the rest of the face. There are typical features such as sebaceous glands, sweat glands, and hair follicles. However, the vermillion is non-keratinized. Specifically, areas in this region are considered non-keratinizing, meaning they lack the typical stratum corneum barrier; they include the labial mucosa and wet surface of the vermillion, ventral tongue, floor of the mouth, soft palate, and buccal mucosa. The mucosa of the oral cavity contains saliva with buffering and solvent action. Susceptibility to allergens and irritants varies among these regions. Many irritants and allergens have classic patterns that can be helpful with making the diagnosis (Table 5.1).

Table 5.1 – Useful patterns of dermatitis

Product	Allergen or irritant	Patterns
Oral cavity		
Dental crowns, fillings/amalgams, dentures, dental braces	Made most commonly from mercury, nickel, gold, and cobalt (allergens)	Buccal mucosa and lateral tongue Lichenoid
Oral hygiene products	Sodium lauryl sulfate (irritant) in toothpastes and mouthwash Flavoring including cinnamon and mint (irritant)	Can be seen on the lips as well as oral mucosa Patchy distribution Toothpaste may show asymmetric involvement of corners of mouth.

Table 5.1 – Useful patterns of dermatitis (*Continued*)

Lips		
Cosmetics	Peppermint oil in lip balm (allergen)	Seen on the upper and lower lips Diffuse distribution
Musical instrument held outward from the lips	Recorder, trumpet	Seen on the upper and lower lips Corresponds with shape of offending product
Musical instrument with a reed or held to the side	Saxophone, clarinet, flute	Lower lip Corresponds with shape of offending product
Habitual oral placement of objects	Pencil, pen, necklace containing nickel (allergen); repetitive trauma (irritant)	Seen on the upper and/or lower lips Corresponds with shape of offending product
Perioral region		
Lip licker dermatitis	Saliva (irritant)	Circumferential irritant dermatitis
Oral hygiene products	See above	See above

Oral cavity

The signs and symptoms of contact dermatitis in the oral cavity are less well defined than those seen with other regions covered in this series. The classic symptomatology of itching and scaling is often absent. Instead, the non-keratinized oral mucosa seems to show a different set of reaction patterns in response to contactants. Lichenoid reactions are a particularly important pattern seen involving the oral mucosa. While oral lichen planus is the prototypical example of this pattern, extrinsic agents such as drugs and contactants should not be overlooked as a potential etiology.[1] Clinically, there may be white reticular patches, erythema, or erosions. The lesions may be asymptomatic or associated with intense burning. The differential diagnosis is broad and often requires a myriad of techniques to finally arrive at the correct diagnosis. A biopsy is typically warranted and helps to rule out things such as connective tissue disease, immunobullous disease and malignancy. Eosinophils seen on histology are helpful in pointing the diagnosis away from lichen planus and favoring an extrinsic driving force such as a drug or contactant.

Historical clues are also extremely helpful in this setting. Recent exposure to dental materials, metals, or plastic sources should be considered significant and patch testing should be initiated. This is particularly important in localized lichenoid dermatitis in close proximity to the suspected oral implant or prosthesis. Areas that should be considered most suggestive for oral contact lichenoid reactions are the lateral tongue and buccal mucosa. These are the areas in closest proximity to amalgams (fillings) and most prosthetic devices.[1] Metals used in dentistry are most often mercury, nickel, gold, cobalt, palladium, and chromium. Sources of exposure to these metals include dentures, braces, crowns, and fillings (amalgams). It is important to search for foreign materials through history and physical exam; and if present, patch testing and removal of offending agent can be of great benefit. Other causes of oral lichenoid contact dermatitis include flavorings (with cinnamon being the classic example) and dental adhesives (acrylates).[2] Allergy to acrylates from dental prostheses may also cause tingling or jaw pain.[3]

One other consideration with regard to contact dermatitis affecting the oral cavity is the so-called "burning mouth syndrome" (BMS). While this disorder is likely a localized dysesthesia with both psychological and neurophysiological components, it may be prudent for some patients to undergo patch testing to help exclude contact dermatitis. It has been suggested that patients with a fluctuating course of BMS may represent a subset of patients in which allergic contact dermatitis is relevant. Unfortunately, only a few patch test studies assessing BMS have been done, and these show mixed results.[4,5]

Oral hygiene products may cause allergic contact dermatitis in either the mucosa of the oral cavity or on the lips.[6-8] Therefore, rashes that involve both the oral cavity and the lips are very suggestive of an allergy to chemicals in mouthwashes, toothpastes, dental floss, and chewing gum. One area of concern is flavorings in toothpastes and oral care products. In general, non-mint-flavored products may be less allergenic. A common offending irritant in these products is sodium lauryl sulfate. In toddlers with skin eruptions in the mucosa of the oral cavity or on the lips, exposure to rubber in pacifiers should also be considered.[9,10] The oral mucosa is frequently exposed to food. Food additives and flavorings may cause mucosal inflammation.

Lips

The lips are often exposed to cosmetic products. In a recent patch test study published by the North American Contact Dermatitis Group, isolated lip dermatitis was determined in 38.3% of patients, most commonly to fragrance mix, balsam of Peru (*Myroxylon pereirae*), and nickel. The most common allergen source was components of cosmetics.[3,11,12] Patch testing is an important step in patients with lip dermatitis. Allergic contact cheilitis may be the result of allergy to chemicals in lip balms, lipsticks, lip glosses, and sunscreens.[12,13] The anatomy of lipstick is surprisingly complex. There are dyes, flavoring agents, sunscreens, and preservatives in addition to the vehicle.[11] A common historical allergen in lip products is castor oil, which is used as a solvent for pigments. Lanolin, another common component in lip products, is used as an emollient and has induced an allergic response in individuals.[12] Cases of postoperative patients reacting to Aquaphor Healing Ointment were shown to react specifically with lanolin alcohol.[14] Benzophenone, a chemical sunscreen found in many lip products and sunscreens, has also been found to be a common allergen.[12] Both allergic contact and allergic photocontact dermatitis may be seen.[15] Patients may sometimes decide to use "natural" products, under the impression the products are free of irritants or allergens. This is a popular misconception, as such products may be contaminated with allergens including bee's wax and associated propolis (also known as bee glue) as well as peppermint.[16] Assessment for natural product lines such as Burt's Bees will help the detection of unsuspecting allergens. As many as one-third of patients with allergic contact dermatitis also had an irritant component contributing to their disease, according to the study by the North American Contact Dermatitis Group.[17]

Exposure to metal lipstick casings or the habitual sucking of metallic objects (pen or pencil) can also be the cause of isolated allergic contact cheilitis to nickel. In these patients, there is often a more focal plaque of chronic dermatitis, which represents the contacted site. Similarly, a focal plaque of chronic dermatitis on the mid-lower lip may be seen in a musician who plays a wind instrument. The allergen may be the mouthpiece itself or the wooden reed.[12,18] There can also be an irritant component to their contact dermatitis from the repetitive trauma to a localized area.

More unique or exotic contactants should also be considered when focal plaques of dermatitis on the lips are present. Things such as musical instruments, pipes, and even blowguns need to be considered (Figures 5.1 and 5.2).[19] Anything that contacts the lips should also be considered, including a significant other or spouse. The transfer of a contactant inadvertently from one person to another (usually a significant other or spouse) has been referred to as consort contact dermatitis. The prototypical vignette is a wife with allergic contact cheilitis to her husband's aftershave.[20]

Perioral region

"Lip licker" dermatitis is an irritant dermatitis that involves the perioral skin.[21-23] Clinically, there is usually a hyperpigmented circumferential symmetric plaque that is red and scaly. A pacifier can trap saliva and create an identical picture in younger children.

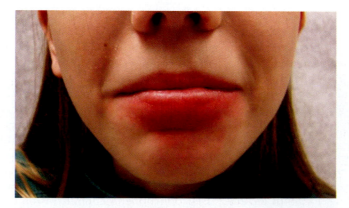

Figure 5.1 – Contact with metal-containing objects such as musical instruments can cause allergic contact dermatitis to the metals or irritant contact dermatitis from the repetitive trauma.

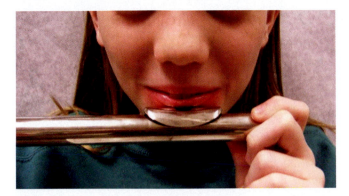

Figure 5.2 – Resulting contact dermatitis from a flute.

While dental products (mouthwash, toothpaste, dental floss, and chewing gum) and medicaments (neomycin, bacitracin, budesonide, tetracaine) are common allergen sources for isolated allergic contact cheilitis, spillover to the perioral skin can also be seen. This is particularly seen in the case of toothpaste-driven allergic contact dermatitis. Both the foaming action of the toothpaste and the movement of the brush contribute to the spread of the toothpaste contactants. Clinically, this can be seen as contact dermatitis at the angles of the mouth. Another helpful clue is that the angles are affected in an asymmetric fashion, with the side on which the toothbrush is held showing more involvement. This is typically the right side in right-handed individuals (Figure 5.3).

Recommendations

When allergic contact dermatitis of the oral cavity, lips, and perioral region is suspected, empiric use of minimally allergenic or hypoallergenic products is recommended. Dermatitis in this area is frequently caused by an allergen, so patch testing can be helpful in determining irritant versus allergic etiologies.[17] Plain petroleum jelly may be used as a lip moisturizer. This is particularly helpful in the case of irritant dermatitis in lip lickers. Individuals should use only plain petroleum jelly and avoid formulations that may have other ingredients. Products such as Vaseline Advanced Formula Lip Therapy will have product labels stating "Active Ingredient: White petrolatum (100%)" portraying pure petrolatum jelly, but such products actually have inactive ingredients such as flavor and fragrance. Fruit flavored toothpastes, such as Tom's of Maine Children's Fluoride-Free Silly Strawberry Toothpaste may be used. For irritant dermatitis of the mouth from sodium lauryl sulfate (SLS), use SLS-free toothpastes such as Sensodyne ProNamel Mint Essence Toothpaste, Burt's Bees Natural Toothpaste, and JASÖN natural toothpastes. For patients who react to acrylates in dentures, prolonged boiling of the dentures has been reported to polymerize residual acrylate monomers, thereby decreasing the allergenicity.[24]

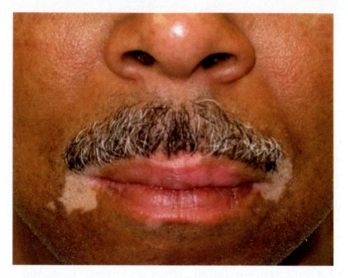

Figure 5.3 – Residual periorificial leukoderma related to contact dermatitis from toothpaste with whitening. This patient demonstrates the classic pattern of accentuation at oral commissures, which is asymmetric, favoring the side where the patient holds the toothbrush.

References

1. Schlosser BJ. Lichen planus and lichenoid reactions of the oral mucosa. 2010. *Dermatol Ther* 23(3):251–267.
2. Tremblay S, Avon SL. Contact allergy to cinnamon: A case report. 2008. *J Can Dent Assoc* 74(5):445–461.
3. Gawkrodger D. Investigation of reactions to dental materials. 2005. *Br J Dermatol* 153(3):479–485.
4. Marino R, Capaccio P, Pignataro L, Spadari F. 2009. Burning mouth syndrome: The role of contact hypersensitivity. *Oral Dis* 15(4):255–258.
5. Dal Sacco D, Gibelli D, Gallo R. 2005. Contact allergy in the burning mouth syndrome: A retrospective study on 38 patients. *Acta Derm Venereol* 85(1):63–64.
6. Ophaswongse S, Maibach H. 1995. Allergic contact cheilitis. *Contact Dermatitis* 33(6):365–370.
7. Kind F, Sherer K, Bircher A. 2010. Allergic contact stomatitis to cinnamon in chewing gum mistaken as facial angioedema. *Allergy* 65(2):274–280.
8. Nadiminti H, Ehrlich A, Udey M. 2005. Oral erosions as a manifestation of allergic contact sensitivity to cinnamon mints. *Contact Dermatitis* 52(1):46–47.
9. Lee PW, Elsaie ML, Jacob SE. 2009. Allergic contact dermatitis in children: Common allergens and treatment. A review. *Curr Opin Pediatr* 21(4):491–498.
10. Militello G, Jacob SE, Crawford GH. 2006. Allergic contact dermatitis in children. *Curr Opin Pediatr* 18(4):383–390.
11. Castanedo-Tardan MP, Zug KA. 2009. Patterns of cosmetic contact allergy. *Dermatol Clin* 27(3):265–230.

12. Orton DI, Salim A, Shaw S. 2001. Allergic contact cheilitis due to shellac. *Contact Dermatitis* 44(4):250.
13. Miura M, Isami M, Yagami A, Matsunaga K. 2011. Allergic contact cheilitis caused by ditrimethylolpropane triethylhexanoate in a lipstick. *Contact Dermatitis* 64(5):301–302.
14. Nguyen JN, Chestnut G, James WD, Saruk M. 2010. Allergic contact dermatitis caused by lanolin (wool) alcohol contained in an emollient in three postsurgical patients. *J Am Acad Dermatol* 62(2):1064–1065.
15. Ortiz KJ, Yiannias JA. 2004. Contact dermatitis to cosmetics, fragrances and botanicals. *Dermatol Ther* 17(3):264–271.
16. Walgrave SE, Warshaw EM, Glesne LA. 2005. Allergic contact dermatitis from propolis. *Dermatitis* 16(4):209–215.
17. Zug KA, Kornik R, Belsito DV, DeLeo VA, Fowler JF Jr, Maibach HI, Marks JG Jr, et al. 2008. Patch-testing North American lip dermatitis patients: Data from the North American Contact Dermatitis Group, 2001 to 2004. *Dermatitis* 19(4):202–208.
18. Mariano M, Patruno C, Lembo S, Balato N. 2010. Contact cheilitis in a saxophonist. *Dermatitis* 21(2):119–120.
19. Onder M, Aksakal AB, Oztas, MO, Gürer MA. 1999. Skin problems of a musician. *Int J Dermatol* 38(3):192–195.
20. Pföhler C, Hamsch C, Tilgen W. 2008. Allergic contact dermatitis of the lips in a recorder player caused by African blackwood. *Contact Dermatitis* 59(3):180–181.
21. Rogers RS 3rd, Bekic M. 1997. Diseases of the lips. *Semin Cutan Med Surg* 16(4):328–336.
22. Zug KA, Kornik R, Belsito DV, et al. 2008. Patch-testing North American lip dermatitis patients: Data from the North American Contact Dermatitis Group, 2001 to 2004. *Dermatitis* 19(4):202–208.
23. de Waard-van der Spek FB, Oranje AP. 2009. Patch tests in children with suspected allergic contact dermatitis: A prospective study and review of the literature. *Dermatology* 218(2):119–125.
24. Koutis D, Freeman S. 2001. Allergic contact stomatitis caused by acrylic monomer in a denture. *Australas J Dermatol* 42(3):203–206.

CHAPTER 6
Neck

Monica Huynh, Michael P. Sheehan, Michael Chung,
Matthew Zirwas, and Steven R. Feldman

Introduction

The neck should be considered among the sites prone to contact dermatitis. Like the eyelids, the thin skin of the neck contributes to the sensitive nature of the region, making it vulnerable to a number of contact allergens. There are many patterns that can be seen in the area that can aid in diagnosis as well as determine the potential allergen (Table 6.1). The neck is often a co-reactor with the face, and the same approach presented in Chapter 3 can be employed when considering the neck. There are three primary categories that should be considered: scalp-applied contact allergens with run-off to the neck, aeroallergens, and directly applied contact allergens.

Scalp-applied allergens are outlined in Chapter 2. It is important to remember that the pre-auricular face, submandibular chin and lateral neck constitute what is

Table 6.1 – Useful patterns for neck dermatitis

Product	Allergen or irritant	Patterns
Aeroallergens		
Fragrance (cologne, perfume)	Balsam of Peru Fragrance mix 1 and 2	Anterior region "Atomizer" sign Patchy distribution
Photoallergen/UV driven		
Sunscreens	Benzophenones	Facial and neck dermatitis Sparing under chin and behind ears
Indirectly contacted allergens		
Nail polish	Tosylamide formaldehyde resin Acrylates	Asymmetric

Table 6.1 – *(Continued)*

Directly contacted allergens		
Jewelry/neck pieces	Nickel	Crescent pattern Anterior neck Corresponds with shape of offending product
Dress shirt/coat collar	Dyes including disperse blue 106 and 124 (increased amounts found in dark clothing) Permanent press clothing containing ethyleneurea/melamine Formaldehyde resin	Encircles the neck Corresponds with shape of offending product
Zippers	Nickel	Patchy distribution Anterior or posterior neck Corresponds with shape of offending product
Necklace clasp	Nickel	Posterior neck Corresponds with shape of offending product
Violin/viola	Exotic woods, metal components, rubber or varnishes	Left side of the anterior neck (just below the angle of the jaw) Patchy distribution Unilateral distribution "Fiddler's neck"

known as the rinse-off pattern, suggesting a scalp-applied allergen that is rinsed off, such as shampoo.

Aeroallergens were discussed in detail in Chapter 3. The neck is typically exposed to the same airborne contactants. In the setting of an aeroallergen-driven dermatitis, the neck may offer the greatest clue—a sharply demarcated cutoff at the shirt collar. Another classic clue found on the neck is what some refer to as the "atomizer sign."[1,2] This is when there is a focal dermatitis located on the anterior neck in the Adam's apple region (Figure 6.1). It is evidence of a focal application of an aerosolized contactant—typically a spray of perfume or cologne. Presence of the atomizer sign is a diagnostic pearl for fragrance-based allergic contact dermatitis.

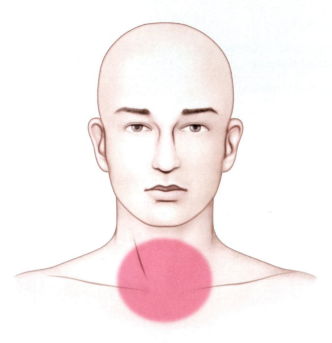

Figure 6.1 – Atomizer sign.

Presentation

Directly applied allergens to the neck can be subdivided into two basic types of contactants: personal care products, including cosmetics and sunscreen, and personal articles such as jewelry and clothing.

A recent article reviewed the results of patch testing to personal care products. Preservatives were the most common allergen to cause a positive patch test result, followed by fragrances.[2] Sunscreens are a unique subset of personal care products that deserve particular consideration. Allergy to the active ingredient in sunscreens appears to be very low (less than 1% of the general population).[3,4] However, sunscreens are involved in a unique niche in the world of contact dermatitis—photoallergic contact dermatitis. While the overall proportion of patients with sunscreen allergy is low, when considering referrals for photopatch testing, sunscreens are the number one photoallergen found to react.[4] Benzophenones are the major class of photoallergenic sunscreens. The primary clue on exam that suggests photoallergic reaction to sunscreens is the photodistribution pattern. Photodermatitis may be mistaken for aeroallergen-driven dermatitis. A helpful distinguishing feature is that the region under the chin and behind the earlobes is typically spared in a photoallergic process.[5]

Nail polish can be considered under the category of personal care products and cosmetics. According to a study on allergic contact dermatitis, the face and neck were the most commonly affected sites for patchy dermatitis secondary to exposure of acrylates in acrylic nails.[4,6,7]

Personal articles include a wide array of items. An allergy to metal in jewelry such as necklaces (Figures 6.2 and 6.3) and earrings (Figure 6.4), and the neck pieces of

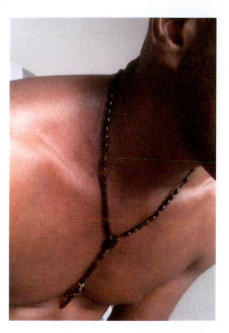

Figure 6.2 – Individual with necklace containing common contact allergen nickel, resulting in allergic contact dermatitis in a necklace distribution.

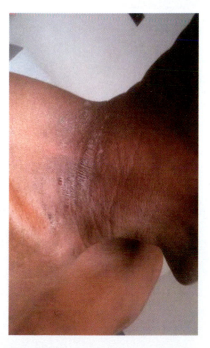

Figure 6.3 – Individual with necklace containing common contact allergen nickel, resulting in allergic contact dermatitis in a necklace distribution.

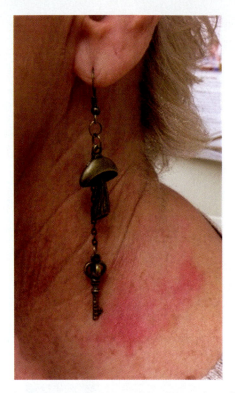

Figure 6.4 – Nickel earring resulting in dermatitis. (Reproduced courtesy of Courtney Orscheln.)

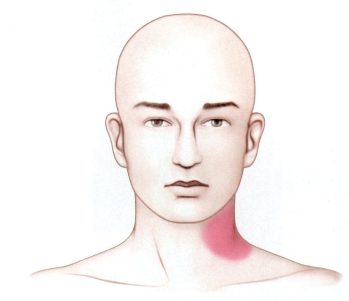

Figure 6.5 – Fiddler's neck.

stethoscopes, may appear as crescent-shaped rashes on the anterior neck.[2,6,7] Wooden necklaces made from exotic woods may also produce an allergic reaction. A more linear band of dermatitis encircling the neck can be a clue that a patient is reacting to the collar of a dress shirt or coat. This may be an irritant reaction if the textile is coarse, such as wool, in a patient with an underlying atopic diathesis. The reaction may also be allergic in nature. The allergen may be primary to the article of clothing, such as textile resins and dyes, or it may be a retained allergen. Retained allergens are most often found in articles that are not frequently washed, such as coats, hats, and shoes. These allergens represent an allergen that has become embedded and retained within the article of clothing. A final pattern is that of posterior neck dermatitis. This pattern may indicate a reaction to dress labels or necklace clasps.[7,8]

Musical instruments can also be considered under personal articles known to cause contact dermatitis affecting the neck. A rash on the left side of the anterior neck (just below the angle of the jaw) in an individual who plays the violin or viola is very suggestive of an allergy to something in the string instrument. This has led to the term "fiddler's neck" being used to describe such presentations (Figure 6.5). These affected individuals often have an allergy to the exotic woods, metal components, or varnishes on the chin rest.[7,9,10]

References

1. Jacob SE, Castanedo-Tardan MP. 2008. A diagnostic pearl in allergic contact dermatitis to fragrances: The atomizer sign. *Cutis* 82(5):317–318.
2. Castanedo-Tardan MP, Zug KA. 2009. Patterns of cosmetic contact allergy. *Dermatologic Clinics* 27(3):265–230.
3. Wetter DA, Yiannias JA, Prakash AV, Davis MD, Farmer SA, el-Azhary RA. 2010. Results of patch testing to personal care product allergens in a standard series and a supplemental cosmetic series: An analysis of 945 patients from the Mayo Clinic Contact Dermatitis Group, 2000–2007. *Journal of the American Academy of Dermatology* 63(5):789–798.
4. Scheuer E, Warshaw E. 2006. Sunscreen allergy: A review of epidemiology, clinical characteristics, and responsible allergens. *Dermatitis* 17(1):3–11.
5. Wolverton S. 2013. Chapter 53. Irritants and allergens: When to suspect topical therapeutic agents. *Comprehensive Dermatologic Drug Therapy*, 3rd edition. Philadelphia: Saunders.
6. Lazarov A. 2007. Sensitization to acrylates is a common adverse reaction to artificial fingernails. *Journal of European Academy of Dermatology and Venereology* 21(2):169–174.
7. Rietschel RL, Fowler JF, Fisher AA. 2001. *Fisher's Contact Dermatitis*, 5th edition. Philadelphia: Lippincott Williams & Wilkins.
8. Sheard C. 1997. *Electronic Textbook of Dermatology, Contact Dermatitis*. Internet Dermatology Society. Available at: http://telemedicine.org/contact.htm. Accessed July 2, 2011.
9. Onder M, Aksakal AB, Oztas MO, Gurer MA. 1999. Skin problems of a musician. *International Journal of Dermatology* 38(3):192–195.
10. Marks Jr JG, Belsito DV, DeLeo VA, Fowler JF Jr, Fransway AF, Maibach HI, et al. 2003. North American Contact Dermatitis Group patch-test results, 1998–2000. *American Journal of Contact Dermatitis* 14(2):59–62.

CHAPTER 7
Hands

Michael P. Sheehan, Monica Huynh, Michael Chung,
Matthew Zirwas, and Steven R. Feldman

Introduction

The hands are a common site for dermatitis. This area remains a diagnostically complex region due to the multifactorial nature of hand dermatitis. Both endogenous and exogenous factors play a role in hand dermatitis.[1] The exact prevalence is difficult to determine because many cases may go unreported. With 20–35% of all dermatitides involving the hands, it is estimated that 2–10% of the general population is affected by hand dermatitis.[2,3]

Contact dermatitis has been reported to be the most common type of dermatitis involving the hands. Several studies have highlighted that hand dermatitis is common among people in occupations involving wet work or exposure to soaps or cleansers. The professions traditionally considered high risk for women are hairdressing and healthcare worker, and for men manufacturing and construction.[3]

Presentation

Developing a differential for potential contactants in hand dermatitis can be challenging. A helpful starting point may be to question the possibility of occupationally or recreationally related causes of hand dermatitis. Risk factors include the use of gloves and chemical exposure. Wet work is also a very important risk factor for hand dermatitis. Exposing the hands to a wet environment daily can lead to maceration of the stratum corneum and impairment of the protective barrier.[4] In these cases, the hands become more susceptible to irritants and potential allergens. According to a cross-sectional analysis by the North American Contact Dermatitis Group, occupational hand dermatitis is frequently related to gloves, bacitracin, preservatives, metals, and fragrance.[3]

Gloves are an example of occupational contact dermatitis due to personal protective equipment (PPE). Gloves are often used in fields such as healthcare, cleaning, and food preparation.[3] The pattern seen with glove dermatitis is somewhat analogous to that seen with shoe dermatitis on the feet. The thinner skin of the dorsal hand and wrists tends to show a patchy dermatitis, while there is relative sparing of the palmar skin. The dorsal forearm may also be involved. Chemicals used in the production of rubber compounds called "rubber accelerators" are considered to be the most common cause of allergic contact dermatitis to gloves. Among the rubber accelerators,

Table 7.1 – Useful patterns for hand dermatitis

Product/allergen or irritant	Pattern
Rubber	
Gloves (latex and rubber additives)	Patchy distribution Favors dorsal hands and wrists
Rubber grip on mechanical pencil/pen	Seen near distal phalanges Corresponds with shape of offending product
Topical medicaments	
Topical antibiotics or corticosteroids	Chronic hand dermatitis refractory to treatment or flaring with treatment
Metals	
Scissors, crotchet hooks	Seen on fingers that hold instrument Corresponds with shape of offending product
Keys, coins, hand-held work tools with metal parts	Corresponds with shape of offending product
Escalator railing, metal bed rail	Seen on palm of hand Corresponds with shape of offending product
Handheld devices (cell phone, computer mouse, etc.)	Seen on palm of hand Corresponds with shape of offending product
Ring	Encircles digit Annular pattern Corresponds with shape of offending product
Miscellaneous	
Artificial nails and/or nail polish	Periungal
Smoking pipe	Most often affects the thumb, index finger, and middle finger (digits 1–3) Varies according to individual preference for holding the smoking pipe

thiurams are the most frequently implicated allergen in glove dermatitis. Carbamates, mercaptobenzothiazole, mixed dialkyl thioureas, chromates, and p-phenylenediamines are other potentially relevant allergens in gloves. An allergy related to rubber components can also be found from many other sources. An isolated and patterned or geometric dermatitis of the hands should initiate a Sherlock Holmes–like approach to obtaining possible contactant history. Some examples of unique rubber contactants affecting the hands include the rubber grip on mechanical pencils and pens, seen as dermatitis near the distal phalanges, and chronic dermatitis of the finger tips in a phlebotomist due to rubber tourniquet use (see Figures 7.1 and 7.2).

Chronic dermatitis of the mid-palm has been termed the palmar grip pattern. This distribution suggests an allergen that is grasped in the palm, such as a computer mouse, cell phone, vehicle stick shift, railing, and cane[7] (Figure 7.3).

Hairdresser dermatitis is another unique form of contact dermatitis secondary to contact with various chemicals found in shampoos, conditioners, and hair dyes

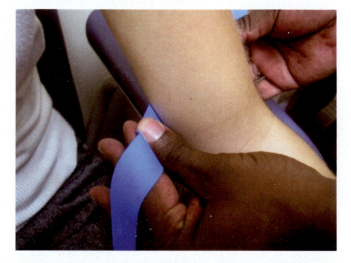

Figure 7.1 – Phlebotomist with rubber allergy from using a standard tourniquet.

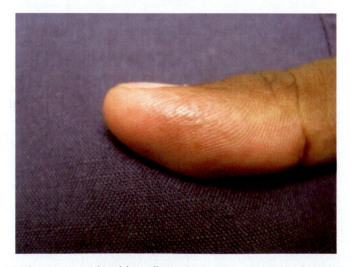

Figure 7.2 – Phlebotomist with rubber allergy from using a standard tourniquet.

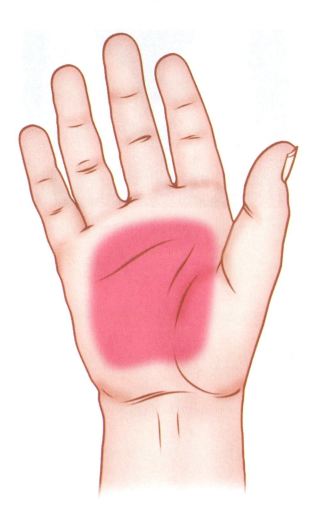

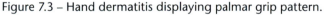

Figure 7.3 – Hand dermatitis displaying palmar grip pattern.

(Figure 7.4). The North American Contact Dermatitis Group has a separate panel of common contact allergens for this occupation as part of their occupation patch test panels (see Chapter 11).

Metal is another common allergen that can affect the hands. While systemic inges-tion of foods high in nickel has been associated with dyshidrosis, hand dermatitis related to metals is more often due to the handling of metal-containing instruments or wearing metal jewelry. Jewelry such as rings (Figure 7.5) may lead to a negative image of dermatitis on the skin that is contacted. Certain occupations are notable for work with metal instruments. A dermatitis localized to the fingers and palm in an individual who works as a hairdresser is very suggestive of an allergy to nickel in nickel-plated scissors.[5] Locksmiths, cashiers, and carpenters are other occupations with frequent exposure to nickel-containing substances such as keys, coins, and hand-held work tools with metal parts.[5,6]

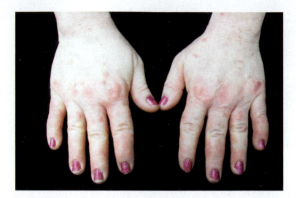

Figure 7.4 – Hairdresser dermatitis from allergen in hair dye.

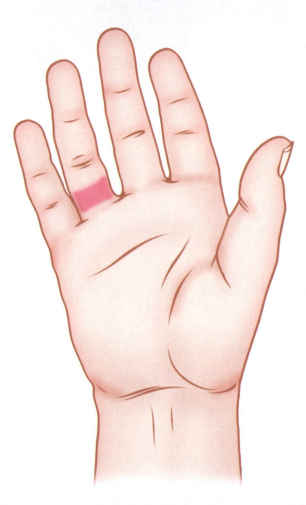

Figure 7.5 – Negative image dermatitis due to a metal ring on the fourth finger.

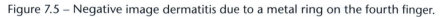

When there is significant inflammation in a periungal distribution of numerous nails, the physician should consider an allergic contact dermatitis to tosylamide form-aldehyde resin nail polish or acrylates in nail glues (Figure 7.6).

Treatment considerations

Irritant contact dermatitis (ICD) is extremely common on the hands and can result from recurrent or prolonged exposure to water or chemicals. The disruption in bar-rier function from ICD allows for potential allergens to penetrate the skin more easily.

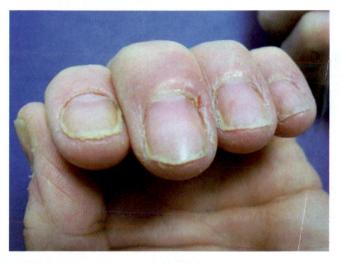

Figure 7.6 – Periungal dermatitis from acrylates in artificial nail glue.

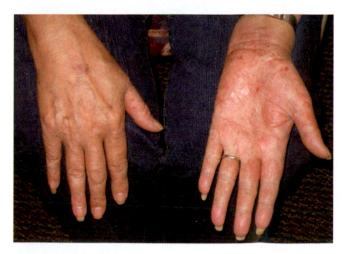

Figure 7.7 – Contact dermatitis medicamentosa sparing the dorsal hands but with a diffuse involvement of the palmar skin and volar wrist.

Wearing proper gloves or minimizing exposure to irritants is essential to providing relief to these patients.

As with all forms of allergic contact dermatitis, avoidance of the causative agent is essential to treatment. This requires investigative work by the patient and physician to determine the underlying cause. When patients are refractory to treatment, consideration should be given to patch testing as well as contact dermatitis medicamentosa.

Contact dermatitis medicamentosa is also important to consider in the evaluation of hand dermatitis. Many cases of hand dermatitis likely begin as xerosis or in adults with atopic dermatitis manifesting as chronic hand dermatitis. This endogenous barrier disruption then sets the stage for hand dermatitis, which becomes secondarily driven by allergic contact dermatitis to the agents utilized for treatment. In these cases there are more patients who demonstrate palmar (Figure 7.7) or diffuse involvement than seen with glove dermatitis. Both over-the-counter and prescription products need to be considered. Bacitracin is a classic example of this.[3] Its use is often seen in the healthcare field and it is also widely applied by patients owing to its availability without prescription. Propylene glycol is another important allergen to consider. It is found in many topical medicaments and is the most common allergen in topical corticosteroid products. It causes both irritant and allergic contact dermatitis. Sorbitan sesquioleate, thiazolinones, lanolin, and formaldehyde-releasing preservatives are other common allergens found in topical corticosteroid vehicles.[1]

References

1. Wolverton SE. 2013. *Comprehensive Dermatologic Drug Therapy*, 3rd edition. Philadelphia: Saunders.
2. Warshaw EM, Ahmed RL, Belsito DV, Deleo VA, Fowler JF, Maibach HI, et al. 2007. Contact dermatitis of the hands: Cross-sectional analyses of North American Contact Dermatitis Group Data, 1994–2004. *Journal of American Academy of Dermatology* 57(2):301–314.
3. Elston DM, Ahmed DF, Watsky KL, Schwarzenberger K. 2002. Hand dermatitis. *Journal of American Academy of Dermatology* 47:291–299.
4. Kiec-Swierczynska M, Chomiczewska D, Krecisz B. 2010. Wet work. *Medycyna pracy* 61(1):65–77.
5. Thyssen JP, Uter W, McFadden J, Menné T, Spiewak R, Vigan M, Gimenez-Arnau A, Lidén C. 2011. The EU Nickel Directive revisited: Future steps towards better protection against nickel allergy. *Contact Dermatitis* 64(3):121–125.
6. Rui F, Bovenzi M, Prodi A, Fortina AB, Romano I, Peserico A, Corradin MT, Carrabba E, Filon FL. 2010. Nickel, cobalt and chromate sensitization and occupation. *Contact Dermatitis* 62(4):225–231.
7. Ghrasri P, Feldman SR. 2010. Frictional lichenified dermatosis from prolonged use of a computer mouse: Case report and review of the literature of computer. *Dermatology Online Journal* 16(12):3.

CHAPTER 8

Extremities

Monica Huynh, Michael P. Sheehan, Michael Chung,
Matthew Zirwas, and Steven R. Feldman

Introduction

The upper and lower extremities are in frequent movement and often make contact with the surroundings. Though contact may be brief or prolonged, this allows upper and lower extremities to be susceptible to many sources of irritants and allergens.

Wrists

Linear rashes encircling the wrist are suggestive of a contactant worn around that region for an extended period of time. Jewelry is a common source and may elicit a reaction to either metal or exotic woods.[1,2] Individuals who wear watches may have a reaction to leather or nickel-containing straps.[3,4] There may be occupationally related rashes in rubber-sensitive individuals who frequently wear rubber bands around the wrist, such as post office workers.[5] In children, exposure to nickel in identification bracelets would also be considered.[6]

Bilateral and symmetrical linear rashes that do not completely encircle the wrists in an individual who works in front of a computer for long periods of time is very suggestive of an irritation or allergic response to keyboard wrist pads and computer wrist rests.[7,8] Exposure to black leather in workout gloves or the dye in the straps (due to the leather or dye) would also be considered.

Forearms

The forearms often rest upon various surfaces, leaving the forearm susceptible to linear rashes with a patchy distribution limited to the medial junction of the volar and extensor forearm surfaces. This presentation would be suggestive of contact dermatitis from worn-out foam, rubber, metal, or Japanese lacquered wood on certain surfaces of furniture such as chairs, sofas, and desktops. Bilateral involvement of the forearms has been reported due to occupational contact dermatitis from ethylene oxide that was used to sterilize green surgical cotton gowns.[9]

Thighs

Although the thighs are often covered by articles of clothing, rashes may occur from the items within the pockets of the clothes. A nummular, or coin-shaped, rash on the anterior thigh in individuals who keep these objects in their pants pockets is very suggestive of an allergy to certain metals (e.g., nickel) in keys and coins.[1,11] The rashes are often unilateral, but bilateral cases have been reported in individuals who use two cell phones simultaneously.[12]

A bilateral nummular rash on the posterior thighs in school-aged children is very suggestive of an allergy to metal in the bolts in certain types of seats. Individuals who made contact between the back of their legs and the metal chair rungs had linear rashes that spanned horizontally across the posterior region of the legs. This pattern below the calves under these circumstances is very suggestive of an allergy to the metal in the chair rungs.

Individuals with chronic leg ulcers are particularly susceptible to polysensitization to topical drugs and antiseptics used to treat their wounds and the surrounding skin.[13,14] In a study of 423 patients with chronic ulcers, 73% had at least one positive patch test. Positive tests were most frequently to balsam of Peru, fragrance, lanolin, and the lanolin derivative Amerchol L101. The duration of the ulcer influenced the patients' sensitization. Frequency of sensitization was 67.5% within 1 year and 79% within 1–10 years.[14]

Scattered arms and legs

One of the most commonly encountered presentations in the clinical setting is a skin rash that presents as a linear streak on the upper and lower extremities. In these cases, a brief history often reveals a recent camping trip or other outdoor activity. This characteristic linear pattern is typical of allergic contact dermatitis due to poison ivy or poison oak.[15-17] The arms and leg can also exhibit sofa dermatitis, as explained in the trunk chapter.

Table 8.1 – Extremities—useful list of allergens and patterns

Product/allergen or irritant	Pattern
Wrists	
Jewelry (bracelets), wristwatches, identification bracelets (children), rubber bands	Encircles wrist Linear pattern Corresponds with shape of offending product
Keyboard wrist pads, computer wrist rests	Patchy or linear distribution Corresponds with shape of offending product
Workout gloves	Patchy or linear distribution Corresponds with shape of offending product

Table 8.1 – (*Continued*)

Forearms	
Wheelchair, chair arms, desktops (worn-out foam, rubber, metal, Japanese lacquered wood)	Volar forearm Patchy distribution Corresponds with sites contacted by offending product
Left arm	
Photoallergens (sunscreens)	May see preference for left arm Dorsal upper extremity May have shirt cutoff
Thighs	
Coins, keys, match boxes	Seen in anterior thigh region (pants pockets) Nummular pattern (coins) Patchy distribution
Metal bolts in seats	Seen in posterior thigh region Nummular pattern Patchy distribution Corresponds with shape of offending product
Metal bar in school chairs (chair rungs)	Seen below the calves Linear or patchy Corresponds with sites contacted by offending product
Arms and legs	
Poison ivy, poison oak	Linear streaky pattern
Furniture (sofa, chairs)	Buttocks, back, dorsal upper thighs, and arms
Fragrances and preservatives (soaps and lotions)	Patchy dermatitis

Asymmetric arm involvement

Photocontact dermatitis occurs when certain allergens produce an allergic reaction upon sun exposure. The left arm is more likely to experience photocontact dermatitis than the right arm, although both may be involved. In North America, the left arm faces the driver's side window, and this sets up the unilateral preference for photocontact dermatitis.[10] Involvement on the dorsal aspects of the arm with sparing of covered regions is a clue to the diagnosis.

References

1. Torres F, Maria das Graças M, Melo M, Tosti A. 2009. Management of contact dermatitis due to nickel allergy: An update. *Clinical, Cosmetic and Investigational Dermatology* 2:39–48.
2. Gomez-Muga S, Raton-Nieto JA, Ocerin I. 2009. An unusual case of contact dermatitis caused by wooden bracelets. *Contact Dermatitis* 61:351–352.
3. Kanerva L, Jolanki R, Estlander T. 1996. Allergic contact dermatitis from leather strap of wrist watch. *International Journal of Dermatology* 35 (9):680–681.
4. Goon AT, Goh CL. 2005. Metal allergy in Singapore. *Contact Dermatitis* 52(3):130–132.
5. Ellison JM, Kapur N, Yu RC, Goldmith PC. 2003. Allergic contact dermatitis from rubber bands in 3 postal workers. *Contact Dermatitis* 49(6):311–312.
6. Tamiya S, Kawakubo YO, Nuruki H, Asakura S, Oazawa A. 2002. Contact dermatitis due to patient identification wrist band. *Contact Dermatitis* 46:306–308.
7. Tanaka M, Fujimoto A, Kobayashi S, Hata Y, Amagai M. 2001. Keyboard wrist pad. *Contact Dermatitis* 44(4):253–254.
8. Yokota M, Fox LP, Maibach HI. 2007. Bilateral palmar dermatitis possible caused by computer wrist rest. *Contact Dermatitis* 57(3):192–193.
9. Kerre S, Goosen A. 2009. Allergic contact dermatitis to ethylene oxide. *Contact Dermatitis* 61:47–48.
10. Levin N. 2003. Rash on the upper arm. *Geriatrics* 58(8):16
11. Rietschel RL, Fowler JF, Fisher AA. 2001. *Fisher's Contact Dermatitis*, 5th edition. Philadelphia: Lippincott Williams & Wilkins.
12. Ozkaya, E. 2011. Bilateral symmetrical contact dermatitis on the face and outer thighs from the simultaneous use of two mobile phones. *Dermatitis* 22(2):116–118.
13. Barbaud, A. 2009. Contact dermatitis due to topical drugs. *Giornale italiano di dermatologia e venereologia* 144(5):527–536.
14. Barbaud A, Collet E, Le Coz CJ, Meaume S, Gillois P. 2009. Contact allergy in chronic leg ulcers: Results of a multicentre study carried out in 423 patients and proposal for an updated series of patch tests. *Contact Dermatitis* 60(5):279–287.
15. Lee NP, Arriola ER. 1999. Poison ivy, oak, and sumac dermatitis. *Western Journal of Medicine* 171(5–6):354–355.
16. Ansar V, Bucholtz J. 2009. Pruritic rash on the arms and legs. *American Family Physician* 79(10):901–902.
17. Levine N. 2001. Vesicles on the extremities: Patients who spend time outside may be especially prone to these lesions in the summer. *Geriatrics* 56(6):18.

CHAPTER 9

Feet

Monica Huynh, Michael P. Sheehan, Michael Chung,
Matthew Zirwas, and Steven R. Feldman

Introduction

The feet are unique among regional contact dermatitides in that they are commonly contained in a microenvironment enclosed by footwear. Depending on the irritant or allergen, the substance can be absorbed by socks and the surrounding shoes. Wearing shoes is a common cultural practice and occurs almost daily for extended periods of time. Since shoes are not routinely washed and socks may be worn for extended periods of time, this allows prolonged exposure to potential irritants and allergens. The combination of shoe and sock contactants plus friction and moisture creates the optimal situation for contact dermatitis to occur. Similar to the hands (Chapter 7), dermatitis involving the thinner dorsal skin is more likely to be contacted in nature. Still, the differential diagnosis for dermatitis of the feet may remain broad.[1] The following are some helpful points to consider in the evaluation of contact dermatitis of the feet.

Presentation

Since sources of contact irritants/allergens causing contact dermatitis of the feet are often more limited, footwear and topical agents are typically at the top of the differential for contactants.[2]

Shoe components have been found to be common allergens in both children and adults.[3] Contact dermatitis due to shoewear can be symmetric or asymmetric, typically starting on the dorsal toes and gradually extending to the dorsum of the foot, sparing the interdigital folds (Figures 9.1 and 9.2). Typical allergens in shoe contact dermatitis include rubber accelerators, leather tanning agents, and adhesives.[5] The most commonly reported rubber-related allergens are the accelerators, including mercaptobenzothiazole (MBT), thiurams, and p-phenylenediamines.[6] More recently, Crocs™ shoes, which have become very popular among physicians and other hospital staff over the past several years, were identified as a source of allergic contact dermatitis on the feet.[7] Other major footwear-related allergens are chromates, p-tert-butylphenol formaldehyde resin (PTBFR), colophony, and paraphenylenediamine (PPD). Chromates, such as potassium dichromate, are used

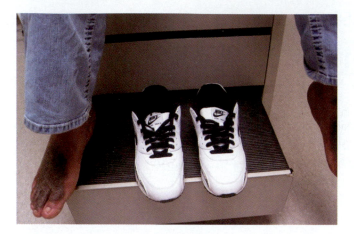

Figure 9.1 – Contact dermatitis due to new pair of shoes.

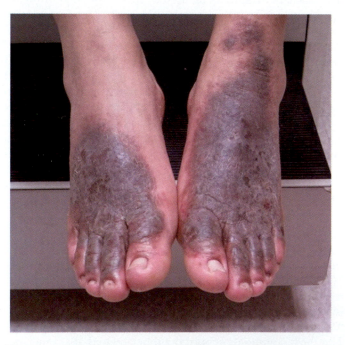

Figure 9.2 – Close-up view demonstrating chronic lichenified plaques of dermatitis on the bilateral dorsal feet. The interdigital spaces and plantar surfaces are spared.

in the leather tanning process, while PTBFR and colophony are common adhesives found in footwear (Table 9.1).[3,4,8]

Important sources of contactants to consider are directly applied personal care products or medicaments. Isolated allergic contact dermatitis of the foot secondary to topical medicaments is most often from topical antibiotics, topical antifungals, or

Table 9.1 – Foot dermatitis—products/allergens and patterns

Product/allergen or irritant	Pattern
Rubber	
Mercaptobenzothiazole (MBT), thiurams, and p-phenylenediamines	Patchy distribution
Leather	
Potassium dichromate	Patchy distribution Seen on dorsum of feet Corresponds with shape of offending product
Adhesives	
P-tert-butylphenol formaldehyde resin (PTBFR), colophony	Patchy distribution
Topical medicaments	
Antibiotics, antifungals, corticosteroids	Diffuse distribution Seen on areas of application, typically dorsal > plantar skin

topical cortisteroids.[1] While topical antibiotics are commonly the inciting allergen, in the case of topical antifungals and topical corticosteroids the patient more often is reacting to the vehicle rather than the active ingredient itself. Expanded patch testing is helpful in determining the precise allergen.

Recommendations

To prevent dermatitis, it is important to:

- Address exacerbating factors such as hyperhidrosis
- Switch patients to minimally or hypoallergenic topical medicaments (Table 9.2)
- Avoid articles that may be contaminated with topical products and allergens such as old socks and shoes

Patients will need to switch shoe types to avoid allergens, such as avoiding leather shoes if there is a potassium dichromate allergy.

Table 9.2 – Hypoallergenic topical antibacterials and antifungals

Antibiotics
Mupirocin
Antifungals
Micatin Cream
Desenex Liquid Spray
Lotrimin AF Cream
Lotrimin Powder/Powder Spray
Tinactin Liquid Spray/Super Absorbent Powder

References

1. Wolverton E. 2013. *Comprehensive Dermatologic Drug Therapy*, 3rd edition. Philadelphia: Saunders.
2. Nedorost S. 2009. Clinical patterns of hand and foot dermatitis: Emphasis on rubber and chromate allergens. *Dermatologic Clinics* 27(3):281–287.
3. Warshaw EM, Schram SE, Belsito DV, DeLeo VA, Fowler JF, Maibach HI, et al. 2009. Shoe allergens: Retrospective analysis of cross-sectional data from the North American Contact Dermatitis Group, 2001–2004. *Dermatitis* 18(4):191–202.
4. Laguna-Argent C, Roche E, Vilata J, de la Cuadra J. 2007. Unilateral contact dermatitis caused by footwear. *Actas Dermosifiliogr* 98(10):718–719.
5. Rietschel RL, Fowler JF, Fisher AA. 2001. *Fisher's Contact Dermatitis*, 5th edition. Philadelphia: Lippincott Williams & Wilkins.
6. Castanedo-Tardan MP, Zug KA. 2009. Patterns of cosmetic contact allergy. *Dermatologic Clinics* 27(3):265–230.
7. Mortz CG, Andersen KE. 2008. New aspects in allergic contact dermatitis. *Current Opinion in Allergy and Clinical Immunology* 8(5):428–432.
8. Rani Z, Hussain J, Haroon TS. 2003. Common allergens in shoe dermatitis: Our experience in Lahore, Pakistan. *International Journal of Dermatology* 42(8):805–807.

CHAPTER 10
Trunk

Laura Sandoval, Courtney Orscheln, Robin Lewallen, and
Steven R. Feldman

Introduction

A diagnosis of allergic contact dermatitis is common and at times fairly clear, though determining the source of the allergen may be more difficult. However, the location and pattern of the dermatitis on the body may provide helpful clues, with classic cases of contact dermatitis often easily identified (Table 10.1). This chapter focuses on contact dermatitis of the trunk.

Presentation

Certain allergens have classical presentations on the trunk. Nickel is one of the most common allergens, and it is often the source of contact dermatitis on the trunk.[1,2] Nickel that exists in belt buckles, buttons on jeans, navel rings, backpack or handbag straps, or clasps of bras will present in a classic distribution with a localized eruption at the site of contact. (Figures 10.1 and 10.2). It can also present as dermatitis on the buttocks or groin/anterior thighs from putting metal objects such as keys, coins, or cell phones in the pockets. Nickel can also cause a unilateral eruption of the left chest in men from objects (such as a cigarette lighter) kept in the left breast shirt pocket. When an allergy on the trunk due to nickel is identified, it may also be present in other classic locations such as the wrist from a watchband or earlobes or neck from earrings. An allergy to deodorants will also present in a classical distribution in the axilla. The most common allergens present in deodorants are fragrance, propylene glycol, essential oils and biological additives, and parabens.[3]

Other common sources of contact dermatitis on the trunk may be less obvious. Preservatives and fragrances are the most common allergens in personal hygiene products such as soaps and moisturizers, as well as in laundry detergents and fabric softeners.[4] In cases of these allergens, the presentation may be a more diffuse eruption with less discrete erythematous papules or eczematous patches and plaques. It may be difficult to distinguish such eruptions from atopic dermatitis or irritant dermatitis. Clothing is a common source of allergens; aside from the detergent or softener being used for washing, the textiles themselves can be the source. The pattern of distribution with textile contact dermatitis is generally increased in areas of friction and perspiration.[5] The dyes used in manufacturing textiles are most frequently

Table 10.1 – Useful patterns for dermatitis of the trunk

Product/allergen or irritant	Pattern
Nickel	
Belt buckle Buttons/clasps Jewelry (necklace, navel ring) Coins/keys	• Often localized to site of contact • Discrete eczematous patches, vesicles may be present
Clothing	

Textiles
  • Dyes
  • Melamine formaldehyde
  • Resins
Detergents/fabric softeners
  • Fragrance
  • Preservatives
  • Dyes
	• Patchy distribution
	• Diffuse eczematous dermatitis

Personal Hygiene Product	

Soaps, moisturizers
  • Preservatives
  • Fragrances/botanicals
Deodorants
  • Fragrance
  • Propylene glycol
	• Patchy distribution
	• Diffuse eczematous dermatitis (except in the case of deodorants where the eruption will be localized to the axilla)

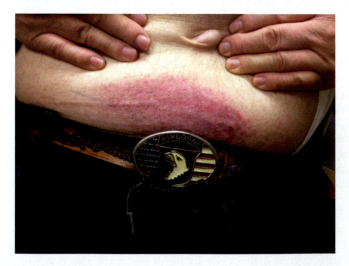

Figure 10.1 – Contact allergy to nickel in belt buckle. (Reproduced by courtesy of Courtney Orscheln.)

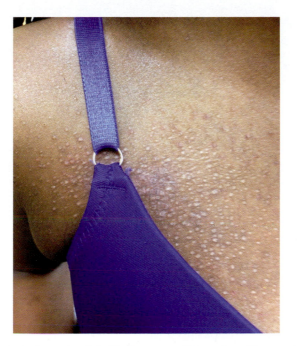

Figure 10.2 – Contact allergy to nickel in bra strap. (Reproduced by courtesy of Courtney Orscheln.)

responsible (average prevalence was highest for disperse blue 106 and disperse blue 124), however, formaldehyde and resins are also common, especially in instances of occupational textile contact dermatitis.[6-8] In one study, nearly 6% of patients who underwent patch testing were reactive to p-phenylenediamine, a black dye which is the traditional textile allergen used in the standard series.[8]

Contact dermatitis on the back can be related to objects that patients lean against when seated. Hexavalent chromium and azo dyes have been identified as allergens present in leather chair and sofa backs, while Japanese lacquer can be the responsible allergen on wood surfaces.[5,9,10]

Recently, an outbreak of "sofa dermatitis" was linked to dimethyl fumarate (DMF), a compound found in both leather and fabric sofas made by a Chinese manufacturer.[10] This allergen was responsible for contact dermatitis, in some cases severe, of the trunk, buttocks, and lower extremity (Figure 10.3). This epidemic of furniture dermatitis was notable in that it led to DMF being selected as the 2011 Allergen of the Year by the American Contact Dermatitis Society.[12]

Recommendations

In cases of allergic contact dermatitis to a known allergen, avoidance of the culprit is recommended. One trick that patients with nickel allergies can try is to cover exposed metal with clear nail polish to prevent exposure to the nickel-containing surface. Jeans with nickel buttons treated with a clear coat of nail polish

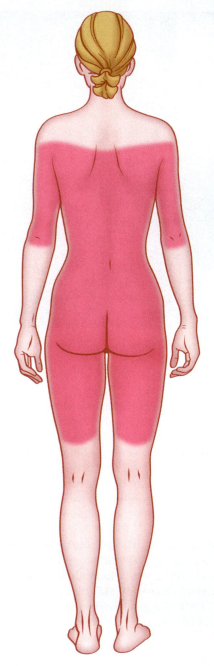

Figure 10.3 – Sofa dermatitis

tested negative with dimethylglyoxime after two washes.[13] There are commercially available nickel-detecting kits that can be used by patients to determine whether nickel is present in a particular item. When contact dermatitis is suspected from an unknown allergen, patients should be advised to avoid common allergens such as fragrances, preservatives, and dyes, and if the allergy persists, patch testing should be recommended.

References

1. Wentworth AB, Yiannias JA, Keeling JH, et al. 2014. Trends in patch-test results and allergen changes in the standard series: A Mayo Clinic 5-year retrospective review (January 1, 2006, to December 31, 2010). *J Am Acad Dermatol* 70(2):269–275.
2. Warshaw EM, Belsito DV, Taylor JS, et al. 2013. North American Contact Dermatitis Group patch test results: 2009 to 2010. *Dermatitis* 24(2):50–59.
3. Zirwas MJ, Moennich J. 2008. Antiperspirant and deodorant allergy: Diagnosis and management. *J Clin Aesthet Dermatol* 1(3):38–43.
4. Wetter DA, Yiannias JA, Prakash AV, et al. 2010. Results of patch testing to personal care product allergens in a standard series and a supplemental cosmetic series: An analysis of 945 patients from the Mayo Clinic Contact Dermatitis Group, 2000–2007. *J Am Acad Dermatol* 63(5):789–798.
5. Brookstein DS. 2009. Factors associated with textile pattern dermatitis caused by contact allergy to dyes, finishes, foams, and preservatives. *Dermatol Clin* 27(3):309–322, vi–vii.
6. Lisi P, Stingeni L, Cristaudo A, et al. 2014. Clinical and epidemiological features of textile contact dermatitis: An Italian multicentre study. *Contact Dermatitis* Jan 7.
7. Malinauskiene L, Bruze M, Ryberg K, Zimerson E, Isaksson M. 2013. Contact allergy from disperse dyes in textiles: A review. *Contact Dermatitis* 68(2):65–75.
8. Wentworth AB, Richardson DM, Davis MD. 2012. Patch testing with textile allergens: The Mayo Clinic experience. *Dermatitis* 23(6):269–274.
9. Patel TG, Kleyn CE, King CM, et al. 2006. Chromate allergy from contact with leather furnishings. *Contact Dermatitis* 54(3):171–172.
10. Ma XM, Lu R, Miyakoshi T. 2012. Recent advances in research on lacquer allergy. *Allergol Int* 61(1):45–50.
11. Susitaival P, Winhoven SM, Williams J, et al. 2010. An outbreak of furniture related dermatitis ('sofa dermatitis') in Finland and the UK: History and clinical cases. *J Eur Acad Dermatol Venereol* 24(4):486–89.
12. Bruze M, Zimerson E. 2011. Dimethyl fumarate. *Dermatitis* 22(1):3–7.
13. Suneja T, Flanagan KH, Glaser DA. 2007. Blue-jean button nickel: Prevalence and prevention of its release from buttons. *Dermatitis* 18(4):208–211.

CHAPTER 11

Anogenital region

Monica Huynh, Michael P. Sheehan, Michael Chung,
Matthew Zirwas, and Steven R. Feldman

Introduction

The anogenital area is susceptible to contact dermatitis due to intrinsic and extrinsic properties. Similar to the eyelid region, the anogenital region is intrinsically prone to irritation and sensitization. Parallels are seen in the fact that both regions have thin epidermal barriers and show a tendency for irritant/allergen retention. The anogenital region differs from other regions in that there is also a high degree of friction, heat, and moisture. These elements contribute to the frequency of several dermatoses in this region (tinea cruris, intertrigo, erythrasma, lichen simplex chronicus).[1] Contact dermatitis in the anogenital region is often secondary to patient- or physician-directed treatment of these conditions, which have lowered the irritant and sensitization threshold.

Presentation

Similar to other regions, it is important to consider both irritant and allergic contact dermatitis. Barrier creams, management of incontinence, and the removal of any harsh irritants are important aspects in controlling anogenital irritant dermatitis. The remainder of this paper will focus on the allergic contact dermatitis (ACD) aspects of the anogenital region.

Data collected by the North American Contact Dermatitis Group has been reviewed with regard to patients with anogenital dermatitis who were referred for patch testing. Of the 575 patients with anogenital dermatitis who underwent patch testing, 347 had isolated anogenital disease. After patch testing, 73 patients were classified as having isolated allergic anogenital dermatitis. In this group, the most common allergens were cosmetics, medicaments, and corticosteroids.[2]

A high index of suspicion is required for the possibility of contact dermatitis medicamentosa in the anogenital region, especially in the setting of a dermatitis that is not responding as expected to conventional therapies. In this setting, particular emphasis should be placed on searching for exposure to topical anesthetics, antibiotics, antiseptics, and preservatives.[1] The rest of the chapter reviews commonly affected areas and their potential allergens (Table 11.1).

Table 11.1 – Anogenital dermatitis—products/allergens and patterns

Product/allergen or irritant	Pattern
Buttocks	
Toilet seats Referred to as "Toilet seat dermatitis"	Seen on buttocks/proximal posterior thighs, Annular pattern, Corresponds with shape of seat.
Diapers Referred to as "Allergic contact diaper dermatitis"	Seen in diaper region, spares bottom of skin folds Subset may mimic the pattern of a cowboy's gun holsters (Lucky Luke dermatitis)
Perianal	
Moistened toilet paper (wet wipes)	Patchy distribution
Vulvar	
Medicaments, condoms, perfumes	Patchy distribution
Penile	
Medicaments	Patchy distribution
Condom	Patchy distribution along the areas covered by the condom

Buttocks

The distribution of the dermatitis on the buttocks can provide many clues to the etiology of the reaction. An isolated annular rash on the buttocks and posterior thighs is nearly pathognomonic for contact dermatitis to a component in toilet seats. Exposure to wooden toilet seats and associated varnish, lacquers, and paints has been reported to result in ACD.[3] This characteristic pattern of allergic contact dermatitis in the buttocks region is known as "toilet seat" dermatitis (Figure 11.1). Toilet seats can also retain irritants and allergens from cleansers. One case report discusses dermatitis due to formaldehyde from a toilet seat, most likely from a public restroom where aggressive cleansers are used to ensure adequate hygiene.[4] Public restrooms and hospitals have been found to be a source of irritant exposure.

Diaper dermatitis affects the area covered by the diaper and is most often irritant in nature. A secondary infection with candida should also be considered. A clue to ACD secondary to diaper components is an eczematous dermatitis that spares the skinfolds and is refractory to conventional therapies for diaper dermatitis. Allergens to consider in this setting include fragrances utilized to provide a pleasant odor to the diaper, coloring dyes, glues, and rubber-related allergens; it is also important to

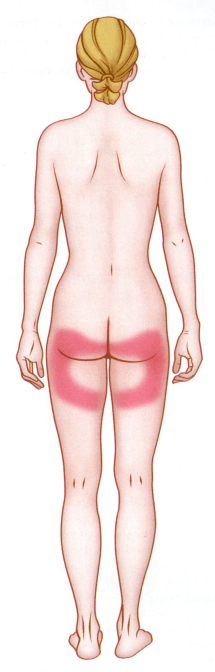

Figure 11.1 – Toilet seat dermatitis.

consider wet wipes, which are often used during the diaper-changing process.[5,6,7] If the pattern of dermatitis favors the hips and lateral buttock, rubber accelerators such as mercaptobenzothiazole should be considered. This pattern has been referred to as the "Lucky Luke" dermatitis and is a subset of allergic contact diaper dermatitis in which the child is reacting to the elastic bands found in disposable diapers.[8,9]

Perianal region

With rashes involving the perianal regions, exposure to perfumed and/or colored toilet paper should be considered.[10] More recently, the use of moistened toilet paper (also commonly referred to as wet wipes) has led to an increase in the number of cases of ACD due to the presence of certain preservatives and fragrances in this consumer product.[11,12]

Vulvar region

The vulvar region is susceptible to the same factors as the general anogenital region. However, estrogen is integral to maintaining the strength and integrity of the vulvar barrier to potential irritants and allergens. Therefore, it is during stages of estrogen deficiency that the barrier is most compromised, thereby leading to susceptibility to both irritant and allergic contact dermatitis. As is always the general rule, the most common type of vulvar contact dermatitis is irritant in nature.[13] Common causes of irritant contact dermatitis include urine, feces, sweat, topical medications, aggressive cleansing, and feminine hygiene products.

Allergic contact dermatitis of the vulva needs to be considered in vulvar dermatoses refractory to treatment. Common causes of allergic contact dermatitis include topical medicaments (such as anesthetics, antibiotics, antifungals, antiseptics, and corticosteroids), latex condoms, and perfumes.[13-15]

Reports have also indicated that flavorings and spices may contribute to contact dermatitis in the vulvar region.[12] This presentation is rare but can be seen in a patient who is reacting to allergens that are excreted in the urine and/or feces. The classic example would be a patient with sensitivity to balsam of Peru, which is a marker not only for fragrance sensitivity but also for flavorings and spices.[16] Therefore it is important to keep in mind that not only locally applied products may lead to contact dermatitis.

Penile region

The foreskin may facilitate the retention and absorption of allergens and eventually play a role in the development of ACD. There is some evidence that circumcision may decrease the risk of inflammatory dermatoses of the anogenital area.[2]

Similar to other areas in the anogenital region, a study by NACDG concluded the most common allergens consisted of fragrances, preservatives, medications, vehicles, and corticosteroids. There should be careful inspection for potential contactants. For example, condoms to increase sexual performance may contain benzocaine gel, which is a known potential contact allergen.

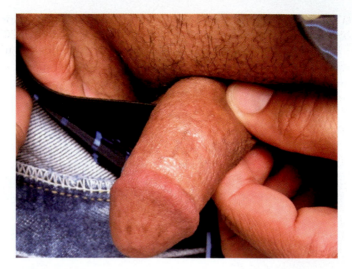

Figure 11.2 – Penile contact dermatitis.

Numerous potential allergens can be found in condoms. Reports indicate ACD has resulted from latex proteins, rubber accelerators, and antioxidants in condoms.[17] Related personal products such as lubricants, dyes, creams, and powders may also contain potential allergens. Figure 11.2 shows a patient with erythema and scaling favoring the corona of glans penis. He had been given a nystatin cream by his primary care physician, which seemed to make the dermatitis worse. The patient's patch test results were positive for both carba mix and ethylenediamine. The initial dermatitis was felt to be from carbamates in the condom; the patient was also reacting to the ethylenediamine in the nystatin cream.

References

1. Wolverton SE. 2012. *Comprehensive Dermatologic Drug Therapy*, 3rd edition. Philadelphia: Saunders.
2. Warshaw EM, Furda LM, Maibach HI, et al. 2008. Anogenital dermatitis in patients referred for patch testing: Retrospective analysis of cross-sectional data from the North American Contact Dermatitis Group, 1994–2004. *Arch Dermatol* 144(6):749–755. doi: 10.1001/archderm.144.6.749.
3. Litvinov IV, Sugathan P, Cohen BA. 2010. Recognizing and treating toilet-seat contact dermatitis in children. *Pediatrics* 125(2):e419–422. doi: 10.1542/peds.2009-2430. Epub 2010 Jan 25.
4. Lembo S, Panariello L, Lembo C, Ayala F. 2008. Toilet contact dermatitis. *Contact Dermatitis* 59(1):59–60. doi: 10.1111/j.1600-0536.2008.01322.x.
5. Lee PW, Elsaie ML, Jacob SE. 2009. Allergic contact dermatitis in children: Common allergens and treatment. A review. *Curr Opin Pediatr* 21(4):491–498. doi: 10.1097/MOP.0b013e32832d2008.
6. Runeman B. 2008. Skin interaction with absorbent hygiene products. *Clin Dermatol* 26(1):45–51. doi: 10.1016/j.clindermatol.2007.10.002.

7. Smith WJ, Jacob SE. 2009. The role of allergic contact dermatitis in diaper dermatitis. *Pediatr Dermatol* 26(3):369–370. doi: 10.1111/j.1525-1470.2009.00934.x.
8. Roul S, Ducombs G, Léauté-Labrèze C, Taïeb A. 1998. 'Lucky Luke' contact dermatitis due to rubber components of diapers. *Contact Dermatitis* 38(6):363–364.
9. DiLandro A, Greco V, Valescchi R. 2002. 'Lucky Luke' contact dermatitis from diapers with negative patch tests. *Contact Dermatitis* 46(1):48–49.
10. Rietschel RL, Fowler JF, Fisher AA. 2001. *Fisher's Contact Dermatitis*, 5th edition. Philadelphia: Lippincott Williams & Wilkins.
11. de Groot AC. 1997. Contact allergy for perfume ingredients in cosmetics and toilet articles. *Nederlands Tijdschrift voor Geneeskunde* 141(12):571–574.
12. Zoli V, Tosti A, Silvani S, Vincenzi C. 2006. Moist toilet papers as possible sensitizers: Review of the literature and evaluation of commercial products in Italy. *Contact Dermatitis* 55(4):252–254.
13. Margesson LJ. 2006. Vulvar disease pearls. *Dermatol Clin* 24(2):145–155, v.
14. Schad K, Nobbe S, French LE, Ballmer-Weber B. 2010. Sofa dermatitis. *Journal der Deutschen Dermatologischen Gesellschaft* 8(11):897–899. doi: 10.1111/j.1610-0387.2010.07386.x.
15. Schlosser BJ. 2010. Contact dermatitis of the vulva. *Dermatol Clin* 28(4):697–706. doi: 10.1016/j.det.2010.08.006.
16. Vermaaat H, Smienk F, Rustemeyer T, Bruynzeel D, Kirtshig G. 2008. Anogenital allergic contact dermatitis, the role of spices and flavour allergy. *Contact Dermatitis* 59(4):233–237. doi: 10.1111/j.1600-0536.2008.01417.x.
17. Blyumin ML, Rouhani P, Avashia NJ, Jacob SE. 2009. Acquiring allergen information from condom manufacturers: A questionnaire survey. *Dermatitis* 20(3):161–170.

CHAPTER 12
Patch testing

Laura Sandoval, Adele Clark, Robin Lewallen, and Steven R. Feldman

Introduction

Identifying the allergen responsible for an allergic contact dermatitis can take a little detective work. First, a thorough history and physical exam must be performed. Areas of involvement on the body may give clues. Inquiring about what the patient does for work and what kind of hobbies he or she has can also be helpful. When possible allergens are identified, patients are often asked to eliminate exposure to these to try to determine or confirm the culprit. However, when this method fails, allergy testing is often recommended. The gold standard for diagnosis of allergic contact dermatitis is patch testing.

The American Contact Dermatitis Society (ACDS) suggests a core allergen series (CAS) that consists of 80 allergens to be included in patch testing.[1,2] A skilled tester, however, can consider various factors to determine the need to test more or fewer allergens, including patient history and the overall clinical picture. Frequency and types of allergens can also vary among communities, so where the patient lives may also be important. Trends in allergenicity are analyzed and reported periodically by the North American Contact Dermatitis Group (NACDG) and several other institutes, including the Mayo Clinic. From the most recent reports, 61–66% of patients have at least one positive reaction on patch testing, with 46% receiving a diagnosis of allergic contact dermatitis.[3,4] A recent overall decline in positive reactions has been reported by both groups.

Methods of patch testing and adverse events

Once it is determined that a patient is an appropriate candidate for patch testing, it is important to educate the patient about the procedure, which can be cumbersome, entailing several visits to the office and requiring the patient to take special care of the patches (for example, depending on the type of patch, patients may be instructed to not bathe for several days to avoid getting patches/test site wet). It is important also to inform patients about potential adverse effects, though serious adverse effects are rare, and set realistic expectations. Most commonly, patients may experience itching at the testing site.[5] Other adverse effects include excited skin syndrome (which can result from a strongly positive test causing hypersensitivity at other sites), a flare-up of existing dermatitis on the skin elsewhere from the testing site, hyperpigmentation, contact leukoderma (a patch-test sensitization that results in a flare-up reaction at least 10 days after initial patch application and which is positive on retesting), and, rarely, anaphylaxis.[6,7] Overall, the benefits of patch testing outweigh the risks when the results lead to a meaningful diagnosis and treatment plan. It may be helpful to develop a patient education handout that provides information on how to prepare for and what to expect from patch testing. The T.R.U.E. Test® website has a handout that provides patients with useful information, such as instructions for before and during testing, possible adverse reactions and how to manage them, and what the results of the test mean (www.truetest.com/9.1%20TT%20QandA_FNL_2013.pdf).[8] A similar useful website for patients is www.mypatchlink.com. A similar handout can be developed to meet your institute's specific needs.

Patch testing should be performed by an experienced tester to ensure accuracy and reliability, both in the method of testing and in the interpretation of results. Prior to testing, it is generally recommended that patients avoid the use of topical and oral corticosteroids for 1–2 weeks. Standard patch testing methods have been adapted; however, there may be variability from institute to institute in the technique, including dilution of allergens, materials used, area of testing, and timing of how long patches are left on and when results are evaluated (Table 12.1).

The majority (68%) of the members of the American Contact Dermatitis Society use the NACDG core series of allergens (using an average of 62 allergens), while only 9% use the Thin-Layer Rapid Use Epicutaneous (T.R.U.E.) Test.[9] The allergens are available as multi-use syringes or dropper bottles and are placed in patch chambers prior to being placed on the patient (Figure 12.1). The T.R.U.E. test is a pre-packaged, ready-to-use patch currently containing 35 allergens that is convenient

Table 12.1 – Patch testing methods

Materials needed: patch trays/chambers,* allergens,* hypoallergenic tape, and permanent marker.
Day 1: Apply patch test, preferably to upper back (Figure 12.2). Secure with tape and outline sites of application with marker. Construct map indicating placement of the allergens. Instruct patient on care of patches/testing sites (for example, some patches must be kept dry while in place).
Day 3 (at 48 hours): Remove patches. Evaluate and score test site. Patient should keep area dry until final reading of test results.
Day 4 (at 72 hours): Test results are reevaluated and scored.**

*Finn chambers (Epitest Ltd, Tuusula, Finland; available in the US from Allerderm Laboratories, Inc.), IQ Chambers™ and allergens (Chemotechnique® Diagnostics; distributed by Dormer Laboratories, Inc.), and allergEAZE® chambers and allergens (allergEAZE; distributed by SmartPractice® Canada)
**Additional readings range from 5 days (96 hours) to 1 week after placement of patches to detect late reactions. If no additional readings are performed after 72 hours, patients should be instructed to note any new positive reactions.

and may be appropriate in certain settings, for example offices where patch testing is not routinely conducted (Table 12.2).[8] While easy to use, the T.R.U.E. may miss up to 27% of positive reactions.[4] A patient's own products may also be tested, appropriately diluted. The reported incidence of patients having a positive reaction to their own products varies from as few as 7% up to about one-third of patients.[10,11] Occupation- or exposure-specific panels of allergens are also available, such as a hairdresser tray or dental tray.

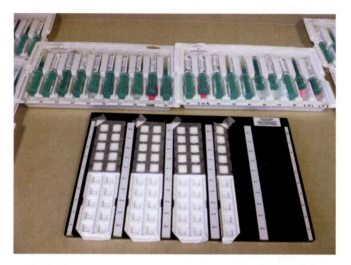

Figure 12.1 – Testing materials including syringes of allergens and chambers (pictured are IQ Ultra Chambers™).

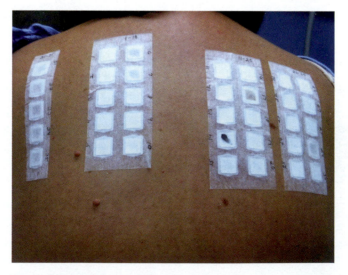

Figure 12.2 – Day 1: Application of patches to upper back.

Table 12.2 – T.R.U.E. test allergens

Panel 1.1	Panel 2.1	Panel 3.1
Nickel	p-tert-butylphenol formaldehyde	Diazolidinyl urea
Wool alcohols		Quinoline mix
Neomycin sulfate	Epoxy resin	Tixocortol-21-pivalate
Potassium dichromate	Carba mix	Gold sodium thiosulfate
Caine mix	Black rubber mix	Imidazolidinyl urea
Fragrance mix	Cl+Me-Isothiazolinone	Budesonide
Colophony	Quaternium-15	Hydrocortizone-17-
Paraben mix	Mercaptobenzothiazole	butyrate
Negative control	p-phenylenediamine	Mercaptobenzothiazole
Balsam of Peru	Formaldehyde	Bacitracin
Ethylenediamine dihydrochloride	Mercapto mix	Parthenolide
	Thimerosal	Disperse blue 106
Cobalt dichloride	Thiuram mix	2-Bromo-2-nitropropane-1,3-diol (Bronopol)

Interpretation of results

Interpretation of patch test results requires both inspection and palpitation of the tested area; again the skill of the person doing the testing is important to ensure reliability. Scoring of the results is generally based on the International Contact Dermatitis Research Group (ICDRG) recommendations proposed in 1970[12,13] (Table 12.3). Irritant reactions can be mistaken for positive reactions, resulting in false positives. Recent reported rates of irritant reactions range between 8 and 15%; however, they appear to be declining compared to previous reports.[3,4] According to the Mayo Clinic, a considerable proportion of reactions were read as mild (macular erythema only), which could potentially lead to false positives or false negatives.[3]

Table 12.3 – Interpretation of patch test results

Score	Result	Presentation
–	Negative	
+?	Doubtful reaction	Faint erythema only
+	Weak	Non-vesicular erythema, infiltration, possible papules
++	Strong positive	Erythema, infiltration, papules, vesicles (Figure 12.3)
+++	Extreme positive	Intense erythema and infiltration and coalescing vesicles, bullous reaction (Figure 12.4)
IR	Irritant reaction	Patchy erythema or papules without infiltration Reaction may not fill the test site

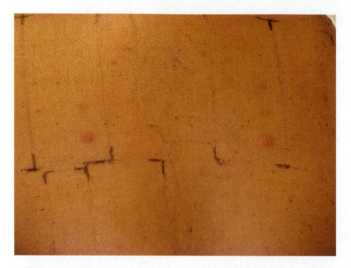

Figure 12.3 – Day 3: Positive reactions.

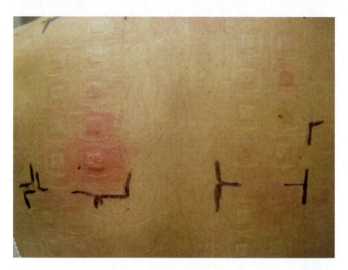

Figure 12.4 – Day 3: Extreme positive reaction to nickel.

Patch testing can be a useful tool in management of contact dermatitis. Identifying specific allergens can help patients avoid future exposure to these. It is important to discuss with patients the relevance of a positive test as well as a negative test. Patients should be counseled on what products contain allergens they tested positive for and alternatives should be recommended, and patients should be taught how to read package labels to avoid known allergens. Written handouts about positive test results can help patients retain this important information. Overall, patch testing can be beneficial for both the diagnosis and treatment of suspected contact dermatitis.

References

1. Schalock PC, Dunnick CA, Nedorost S, et al. 2013. American Contact Dermatitis Society core allergen series. *Dermatitis* 24(1):7–9.
2. Lee J, Warshaw E, Zirwas MJ. 2011. Allergens in the American Contact Dermatitis Society core series. *Clin Dermatol* 29(3):266–272.
3. Wentworth AB, Yiannias JA, Keeling JH, et al. 2013. Trends in patch-test results and allergen changes in the standard series: A Mayo Clinic 5-year retrospective review (January 1, 2006, to December 31, 2010). *J Am Acad Dermatol* 70(2):269–275.
4. Warshaw EM, Belsito DV, Taylor JS, et al. 2013. North American Contact Dermatitis Group patch test results: 2009 to 2010. *Dermatitis* 24(2):50–59.
5. Kunkeler L, Bikkers SC, Bezemer PD, et al. 2000. (Un)usual effects of patch testing? *Br J Dermatol* 143(3):582–586.
6. Devos SA, van der Valk PG. 2002. Epicutaneous patch testing. *Eur J Dermatol* 12(5):506–513.
7. Cronin E. 1980. *Contact Dermatitis*, pp. 1–19. Edinburgh, London, and New York: Churchill Livingstone.
8. T.R.U.E. Test. http://www.truetest.com/ (accessed December 16, 2013).
9. Schleichert RA, Hostetler SG, Zirwas MJ. 2010. Patch testing practices of American Contact Dermatitis Society members. *Dermatitis* 21(2):98–101.
10. Slodownik D, Williams J, Frowen K, et al. 2009. The additive value of patch testing with patients' own products at an occupational dermatology clinic. *Contact Dermatitis* 61(4):231–35.
11. Uter W, Balzer C, Geier J, Frosch PJ, Schnuch A. 2005. Patch testing with patients' own cosmetics and toiletries: Results of the IVDK, 1998–2002. *Contact Dermatitis* 53(4):226–33.
12. Wilkinson DS, Fregert S, Magnusson B, et al. 1970. Terminology of contact dermatitis. *Acta Derm Venereol* 50(4):287–292.
13. Fregert S. 1981. *Manual of Contact Dermatitis*, 2nd edition. Copenhagen: Munksgaard.

CHAPTER 13
Treatment considerations

Farah Moustafa and Robin Lewallen

The goal of treatment of allergic contact dermatitis (ACD) is to minimize associated morbidity and avoid complications. The mainstay of treatment of allergic contact dermatitis is topical corticosteroids. Successful treatment outcomes, however, depend on identification and avoidance of causative allergens. In the initial approach to managing patients with suspected ACD, it is best to advise patients to broadly and non-selectively avoid potential allergens until diagnostics such as patch testing can identify the specific allergens. Figures 13.1 and 13.2 show a patient with ACD before and after treatment.

Topical corticosteroids

Topical corticosteroids (TCS) are the mainstay of treatment in patients with allergic contact dermatitis. The strength of TCS varies on body site affected (Table 13.1).

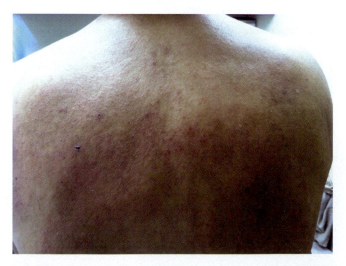

Figure 13.1 – Middle-aged Indian man with a several-month history of contact dermatitis. Patch testing confirmed allergies to lanolin alcohol, balsam of Peru, and propylene glycol.

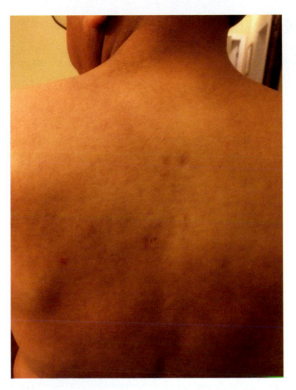

Figure 13.2 – Resolution of contact dermatitis of the shoulder after treatment with systemic and topical steroids for one week. There is residual hyperpigmentation.

Table 13.1 – Recommendations for TCS selection based on anatomical location of dermatitis

Body site	Recommended corticosteroid strength	Examples
Extremities (hands, feet)*	Class 1 (super potent)	Clobetasol propionate 0.05% Halobetasol propionate 0.05%
Intertriginous sites Face**	Class 6 (mild), 7 (least potent)	Class 6 Desonide 0.05% Class 7 Hydrocortisone 2.5%
Flexural areas	Class 5 (mid-potency), 6 (mild), 7 (least potent)	Class 5 Triamcinolone acetonide 0.1% Class 6 (see above) Class 7 (see above)

*Avoid prolonged (greater than 2–3 weeks) daily use on the nails to avoid osteonecrosis.
**Avoid use on eyelids and close proximity to eyes (for periocular area see section on immunomodulators).

Allergic contact dermatitis to topical corticosteroids

Although paradoxical, patients can in fact develop allergic contact dermatitis to TCS themselves. This is often hard to diagnose, as a hypersensitivity to the TCS is confounded by the underlying disease process and requires a strong clinical suspicion. Often, the skin condition worsens after treatment with a TCS. The reaction is due to either the steroid itself or added preservatives. Incidence of steroid hypersensitivity is reported to be between 0.5 and 5%.[1] Hypersensitivity reactions to steroid molecules are divided into two categories: immediate reactions, typically occurring within one hour of drug administration, and delayed reactions, which occur more than an hour after drug administration. The delayed reactions most commonly present as allergic contact dermatitis. Evaluation and management of these patients, like patients with other forms of allergic contact dermatitis, depends on patch testing. This helps identify not only which TCS the patient cannot tolerate, but also other classes of steroids that are not cross-reactive and that patients can tolerate.

Corticosteroids are divided into four classes on the basis of structure and cross-reactivity pattern: class A (hydrocortisone type), B (triamcinolone acetonide type), C (betamethasone type), and D. Class D is divided into 2 subclasses: D1 (betamethasone dipropionate type) and D2 (methylprednisolone aceponate type). During patch testing for identification of a steroid allergy, representative molecules from each class are used as screening markers for allergy to that specific class.[2] Of all classes, Class A steroids most commonly cause a positive patch reaction. Class C positive reactions are very rare.[3] C-16 methyl corticosteroids (betamethasone dipropionate, clobetasol propionate, diflorasone diacetate, fluticasone propionate, mometasone furoate, desoxymethasone) are far less allergenic than non-methylated molecules (hydrocortisone, hydrocortisone-21-butyrate, hydrocortisone-17-butyrate).[4]

Not only can the steroid molecules themselves be allergens, the vehicles in which they are delivered can also cause allergic contact dermatitis. The most common allergen in TCS is propylene glycol. This colorless, clear viscous liquid is present in 64% of

Table 13.2 – Allergic contact dermatitis to TCS determined via patch testing

Steroid class	Screening agent	Cross reactions
Class A	Tixocortol-21-pivalate	Cross reacts with D2
Class B	Budesonide and triamcinolone acetonide	Budesonide specifically cross reacts with D2
Class C	None	None
Class D1	Clobetasol-17-propionate	None
Class D2	Hydrocortisone-17-butyrate	Cross reacts with Class A and budesonide

Certain screening agents are used to determine the class of allergy; cross-reactivity between classes is possible.

Table 13.3 – Propylene glycol-free topical corticosteroids available in the United States

Brand name (active ingredient)	O	G	C	L	S	T
DesOwen 0.05% (betamethasone valerate)	X					
Topicort 0.05% (desoximetasone)	X	X	X			
Topicort 0.25% (desoximetasone)	X				X	
Synalar 0.025% (fluocinolone acetonide)	X					
Cordran 0.05% (flurandrenolide)				X		X
Halog 0.1% (halcinonide)	X					
Pramosone 1%, 2.5% (hydrocortisone acetate)				X		
Pramosone E 2.5% (hydrocortisone acetate)			X			
Locoid 0.1% (hydrocortisone butyrate)			X	X		
Kenalog (triamcinolone acetonide)					X	

O = ointment, G = gel, C = cream, L = lotion, S = solution, T = tape
Generic propylene glycol-free formulations of triamcinolone and clobetasol are available in the United States and vary based on manufacturer.

TCS preparations. Because it is present in so many products, it is important to know alternatives to offer patients with a propylene glycol allergy (Table 13.3).[5] Generic propylene-glycol-free formulations of triamcinolone and clobetasol are available in the United States. These vary based on the manufacturer, so it is important to specify "propylene glycol free" in the instructions to the pharmacy. Other allergens found in topical corticosteroids are sorbitan sesquioleate, formaldehyde-releasing preservatives, parabens, methylchloroisothiazolinone, lanolin, and fragrance.[3] When there is a question about the ingredients it is best to have the patient bring in the products that they are using, including the packaging for a list of ingredients, or to refer to http://dailymed.nlm.nih.gov/ to look up the product prior to prescribing a potentially offending agent.

Topical immunomodulators

This class includes calcineurin inhibitors such as tacrolimus and pimecrolimus. Although topical corticosteroids remain the drug of choice for the initial treatment of uncomplicated ACD, there are several instances where the use of topical immunomodulators can offer an advantage over topical corticosteroids. A clinically important indication for use of topical immunomodulators is for ACD involving the face and periorbital area. Use of topical immunomodulators as "steroid-sparing therapy" in these areas protects the patient from TCS side effects, including skin atrophy, glaucoma, and cataracts.[6] Other indications for use of this class are ACD resistant to topical corticosteroids or treatment of ACD in a patient who has a topical corticosteroid allergy.[7,8] Of note, tacrolimus is propylene glycol free (contains propylene carbonate), whereas pimecrolimus does contain propylene glycol.

Systemic steroids

Systemic corticosteroids are used in cases of severe acute contact dermatitis, or extensive area of involvement (>20% body surface area), or for quicker relief in the involvement of sensitive areas.[9] They are often used in the case of poison ivy ACD, as the presentation is often acute and severe. Treatment with oral corticosteroids usually involves a two-week taper with a prednisone starting dose of 1 mg/kg. Steroids should be tapered down to prevent rebound dermatitis.

Systemic immunomodulators

These drugs include methotrexate, azothioprine, mycophenolate and cyclosporine. They are rarely used and reserved for patients with severe and chronic disease or cases where allergen avoidance is not possible.[10]

Low allergen topical medications

Patients with a known allergy to commonly used topical medicaments for acne, rosacea, seborrhea, psoriasis, or actinic keratoses can be particularly challenging to treat. Having a high level of suspicion for irritant or allergic contact dermatitis from topical medications and good understanding of the best agents to use in these patients is important in the proper management of these patients (Table 13.4).

Irritant contact dermatitis

As with allergic contact dermatitis, avoidance of causal agents is key in treatment of irritant contact dermatitis. Most irritant contact dermatitis involves the hands, and therefore hand protection (gloves) is a mainstay of treatment.[11] Gloves should be worn for wet or dirty tasks at the workplace or at home. Many types of gloves exist and offer specific protection based on the chemical and irritant exposure (Table 13.5).[12] Gloves should be used for duration of exposure, but for the shortest time possible to limit sweating and potential irritation. Thin cotton gloves should be worn under tight-fitting gloves and changed as soon as they become damp. In addition to avoidance and skin protection, active treatment may reduce existing inflammation and restore the epidermal barrier (Table 13.6).

Table 13.4 – Minimally or hypoallergenic prescription topical agents

	Medication	Allergen(s)
Acne	Acanya Gel	PG
	Atralin Gel	Parabens, BHT
	Benzaclin Gel	None
	Differin Gel (0.1%, 0.3%)	Parabens, PG
	Differin Cream	Parabens
	Duac Gel	None
	Retin-A Micro Gel (0.1%, 0.04%)	PG, BHT
	Tazorac Gel	BHA, BHT
	Tazorac Cream	None
Rosacea	Finacea Gel	PG
	Metrogel	Parabens, PG
Psoriasis	Dovonex Cream	Diazolidinyl urea
	Taclonex Ointment	None
	Vectical	None
Seborrhea	Promiseb	Propyl gallate
	Tersifoam	Parabens, PG
	Xolegel	BHT, PG
Actinic keratosis	Solaraze Gel	None
	Zyclara	Parabens
	Efudex	Parabens, PG

PG = propylene glycol; BHT = butylated hydroxytoluene; BHA = butylated hydroxyanisole

Table 13.5 – List of protective gloves based on hazardous exposure

Exposure	Gloves
Microorganisms	NRL, thermoplastic elastomer
Pharmaceuticals	NRL

(Continued)

Table 13.5 – *(Continued)*

Disinfectants	NRL, PVC, PE, EMA
Detergents	NRL, PE, neoprene, PVC, nitrile
Corrosives	NRL, PE, PVC, neoprene, butyl rubber, 4H gloves
Machining oils	NRL, PVC, nitrile, neoprene, 4H glove
Solvents	NRL, PE, PVC, nitrile, neoprene, butyl rubber, 4H gloves

NRL = natural rubber latex; PVC = polyvinyl chloride; PE = polyethylene

Table 13.6 – Summary of treatment recommendations for irritant contact dermatitis

Treatment	Recommendations for use	How to use	Data supporting use
Topical corticosteroid	Steroids are used in cases of severe acute ICD or chronic ICD	Apply 1–2 times daily for 2–4 weeks Steroid selection is based on anatomic site of involvement and severity See Table 13.1 for suggestions	Efficacy is unproven and use in treatment is still controversial[13] In some cases, corticosteroid use can induce ICD[14]
Emollients or moisturizers	Can be helpful in all patients with ICD	Because they offer a protective barrier only when on the skin, they should be applied frequently throughout the day, particularly after hand washing and work Main types: • Occlusive: petroleum, lanolin, ceramides, silicones • Humectant: glycerin, sorbital, lactic acid, alpha hydroxy acids, urea • Emollient: cholesterol • Fatty acids Barrier: dimethicone, liquid paraffin, aluminum chlorohydrate	Moisturizers are sometimes effective for preventing and treating irritant dermatitis.[15] Barrier creams can help prevent ICD in certain occupations[16] Some moisturizers contain irritants

References

1. Matura M, Goossens A. 2000. Contact allergy to corticosteroids. *Allergy* 55(8):698–704.
2. Jacob SE, Steele T. 2006. Corticosteroid classes: A quick reference guide including patch test substances and cross-reactivity. *J Am Acad Dermatol* 54(4):723–727.
3. Coloe J, Zirwas MJ. 2008. Allergens in corticosteroid vehicles. *Dermatitis* 19(1):38–42.
4. Baeck M, Chemelle JA, Goossens A, Nicolas JF, Terreux R. 2011. Corticosteroid cross-reactivity: clinical and molecular modelling tools. *Allergy* 66(10):1367–1374.
5. Daily Med. RSS. N.p., n.d. Web. 2 Jan. 2014 (http://dailymed.nlm.nih.gov).
6. Hengge UR, Ruzicka T, Schwartz RA, Cork MJ. 2006. Adverse effects of topical glucocorticosteroids. *J Am Acad Dermatol* 54(1):1–15.
7. Katsarou A, Makris M, Papagiannaki K, Lagogianni E, Tagka A, Kalogeromitros D. 2012. Tacrolimus 0.1% vs mometasone furoate topical treatment in allergic contact hand eczema: A prospective randomized clinical study. *Eur J Dermatol* 22(2):192–196.
8. Vatti RR, Ali F, Teuber S, Chang C, Gershwin ME. 2013. Hypersensitivity reactions to corticosteroids. *Clin Rev Allergy Immunol* April.
9. Beltrani VS, Bernstein L, Cohen DE, et al. 2006. Contact dermatitis: A practice parameter. *Ann Allergy Asthma Immunol* 97(3 Suppl 2):S1–38.
10. Verma KK, Mahesh R, Srivastava P, Ramam M, Mukhopadhyaya AK. 2008. Azathioprine versus betamethasone for the treatment of parthenium dermatitis: A randomized controlled study. *Indian J Dermatol Venereol Leprol* 74(5):453–457.
11. Bourke J, Coulson I, English J. 2009. Guidelines for the management of contact dermatitis: An update. *British Journal of Dermatology* 160:946–954.
12. Mellstrom GA, Bowman A. 2000. Protective gloves. *Handbook of Occupational Dermatology* 416–435.
13. Levin C, Zhai H, Bashir S, Chew AL, Anigbogu A, Stern R, Maibach H. 2001. Efficacy of corticosteroids in acute experimental irritant contact dermatitis. *Skin Res Technol* 7(4):214–218.
14. Clemmensen A, Andersen F, Petersen TK, Hagberg O, Andersen KE. 2011. Applicability of an exaggerated forearm wash test for efficacy testing of two corticosteroids, tacrolimus and glycerol, in topical formulations against skin irritation induced by two different irritants. *Skin Res Technol* 17(1):56–62.
15. Yokota M, Maibach HI. 2006. Moisturizer effect on irritant dermatitis: An overview. *Contact Dermatitis* 55(2):65–72.
16. Bauer A, Schmitt J, Bennett C, Coenraads PJ, Elsner P, English J, Williams HC. 2010. Interventions for preventing occupational irritant hand dermatitis. *Cochrane Database Syst Rev* June 16; (6):CD004414.

Quick reference

Topical corticosteroids by class strength and structure			
Class strength	**Class structure**		
Class 1 (Super Potent)	Class D1		
	Betamethasone diproprionate 0.05% (G, O, L) Clobetasol proprionate 0.05% (C, O, G, S, F) Diflorasone diacetate 0.05% (O)		
Class 2 (High Potency)	Class B	Class C	Class D1
	Amcinonide 0.1% (O, L, C) Budesonide 0.025% (C) Fluocinonide 0.05% (C, O, G, S) Halcinonide 0.1% (C, O, S)	Desoximetasone 0.25% (C), 0.05% (G)	Betamethasone dipropionate 0.05% (O, C) Betamethasone valerate 0.1% Diflorasone diacetate 0.05%
Class 3 (Upper Mid-Strength)	Class B	Class D1	
	Amcinonide 0.1% (L) Fluocinonide 0.05% Triamcinolone acetonide 0.1% (C, O) Triamcinolone diacetate 0.1% (C, O)	Betamethasone dipropionate 0.05% (C) Betamethasone valerate 0.1% (O) Clobetasone butyrate 0.05% Diflorasone diacetate 0.05% (C) Fluticasone propionate 0.005% (O) Mometasone furoate 0.1% (O)	

Class 4 (Mid-Strength)	Class B	Class C	Class D1	Class D2
	Amcinonide 0.1% (C) Fluocinolone acetonide 0.01%, 0.025% (O) Halcinonide 0.025% (C) Triamcinolone acetonide 0.1% (O) Triamcinolone diacetate 0.1% (O)	Clocortolone pivalate 0.1% (C) Desoximetasone 0.05% (C)	Betamethasone valerate 0.12% (F) Clobetasone butyrate 0.05% Mometasone furoate 0.1% (C, L)	Hydrocortisone valerate 0.2% (O)

Class 5 (Lower Mid-Strength)	Class B	Class D1	Class D2
	Desonide 0.05% (O) Fluocinolone acetonide 0.025% (C) Triamcinolone acetonide 0.1% (C), 0.025% (O, L) Triamcinolone diacetate 0.1% (C)	Betamethasone dipropionate 0.05% (L) Betamethasone valerate (C, L) Fluticasone propionate 0.05% (C)	Hydrocortisone buteprate 0.1% (C, O, S) Hydrocortisone butyrate 0.1% (C, O, S) Hydrocortisone valerate 0.2% (C) Prednicarbate 0.1% (C)

Class 6 (Low Potency)	Class B	Class D1
	Desonide 0.05% (C, F) Fluocinolone acetonide 0.01% (C, S) Triamcinolone acetonide 0.025% (C) Triamcinolone diacetate 0.025% (C)	Alclometasone dipropionate 0.05% (C, O) Betamethasone valerate 0.1% (C)

Class 7 (Least Potent)	Class A
	Hydrocortisone Hydrocortisone acetate Methylprednisolone, prednisolone Tixocortol pivalate

Legend: C=Cream, G=Gel, L=Lotion, O=Ointment, S=Solution, F=Foam

Adapted from Jacob SE, Steele T. Corticosteroid classes: a quick reference guide including patch test substances and cross-reactivity. *J Am Acad Dermatol* 2006;54:723–727.

Index

Index

Index

Index